The NLP Diet

Teach® Yourself

The NLP Diet: Think Yourself Slim for Good

Jeff Archer

Hodder Education
338 Euston Road, London NW1 3BH.

Hodder Education is an Hachette UK company

First published in UK 2011 by Hodder Education

First published in US 2011 by The McGraw-Hill Companies, Inc.

This edition published 2011.

British Library Cataloguing in Publication Data: a catalogue record
for this title is available from the British Library.

Library of Congress Catalog Card Number: on file.

10 9 8 7 6 5 4 3 2 1

The publisher has used its best endeavours to ensure that any
website addresses referred to in this book are correct and active at
the time of going to press. However, the publisher and the author
have no responsibility for the websites and can make no guarantee
that a site will remain live or that the content will remain relevant,
decent or appropriate.

The publisher has made every effort to mark as such all words
which it believes to be trademarks. The publisher should also
like to make it clear that the presence of a word in the book,
whether marked or unmarked, in no way affects its legal status as
a trademark.

Every reasonable effort has been made by the publisher to trace the
copyright holders of material in this book. Any errors or omissions
should be notified in writing to the publisher, who will endeavour
to rectify the situation for any reprints and future editions.

Hachette UK's policy is to use papers that are natural, renewable
and recyclable products and made from wood grown in sustainable
forests. The logging and manufacturing processes are expected to
conform to the environmental regulations of the country of origin.

www.hoddereducation.co.uk

Typeset by MPS Limited, a Macmillan Company.

Printed in Great Britain by CPI Cox & Wyman, Reading.

Contents

About the author

The objective of this book is simple. To enable you to achieve long-term weight loss with the help of Neuro-Linguistic Programming techniques.

I first discovered Neuro-Linguistic Programming (NLP) a number of years ago when I was working as a freelance personal trainer. Having gained my initial qualifications and spent a few months working with a number of clients, I began to wonder why some of these clients experienced quicker results than others when it came to losing weight. The people I was working with all shared similar lifestyle routines. All were successful professionals with either a busy family life or a full social diary, and the way I was working with each of them was fairly consistent. So what was causing the differences in their results?

I began to analyse my styles of teaching, and my methods of communicating the knowledge I had to each of these individuals. At the same time I thought it might be useful to understand more about what motivates people to see if I could identify any personality traits or lifestyle influences that would help me find more effective ways to inspire every single one of my clients. I began researching the psychology of successful people and the behaviour and characteristics that made those people stand out in their chosen field. The more I read, the more I came across information that led back to techniques and explanations rooted in NLP.

I wanted to know more about NLP and during my research I read many definitions of NLP but, even then, I was still unsure of exactly what NLP was. What attracted me to the ideas I was encountering was that I could quickly think of practical applications for what I was reading; I could call to mind specific examples from previous work experiences where being in possession of the knowledge I was gaining would have helped a great deal. I could also recognize many situations where my current clients would now benefit from a new approach involving the techniques I was finding out about.

I decided to experiment with some of these techniques and try them out on my clients. The results amazed me and impressed my clients. This book will explain many of the NLP techniques that I applied to help my clients lose weight and stay slim for good, and will give you the opportunity to try them out for yourself. I hope you're ready for some amazing results!

In one minute

This is a book for anyone who has ever attempted to lose weight. There are many diet plans on the market but many of them seem to have a 'sell-by' date for each person who tries them. The reason for this is that each of these diet plans invariably requires a great deal of conscious thought and effort. To stick to the diet, you have to make detailed plans and behave in a way that may not come naturally to you. After a while it's just easier to return to old behaviour patterns, even if this means that your weight management plans suffer.

NLP suggests a number of approaches that can fundamentally change the way you think about losing weight. This book will help you understand more about why you want to lose weight and explain how you can use past experiences to achieve more effective results in the future.

As you'd expect with a book that promises such dramatic results, there will be plenty of opportunities for you to contemplate your personal situation and devise new strategies that will work for you. You'll be developing your own unique recipe for success. *The NLP Diet* is not just a book to read and move on from; it's a text that will change the way you think for good.

Believe in yourself

In this chapter you will learn:
- *how NLP can help you stay slim for good*
- *how to challenge limiting weight-management beliefs*
- *how to update your belief system to ensure quick weight loss.*

What is Neuro-Linguistic Programming?

Neuro-Linguistic Programming (NLP) is many things to many people. There are a number of possible definitions and many of them are included in the very useful, *Essential NLP* by Steve Bavister and Amanda Vickers. A definition featured there which encapsulates the essence of NLP, particularly when it comes to applying it to weight loss, is as follows:

> *[NLP is]…a system for describing, restructuring and transforming a person's meaning and cognitive understanding of the world they live in.*

Put simply, NLP techniques help you understand how you currently interpret the world around you and how it shapes what you think and feel, and offer suggestions on ways in which you can change your thoughts and behaviour to become more effective with whatever you are trying to achieve. As a title, Neuro-Linguistic Programming is a bit of a mouthful but it covers the essential components of the discipline. 'Neuro' applies to the way you think, 'linguistic' to the language you use, and 'programming' to the ways in which you set yourself up to operate in the world around you.

NLP has many applications and the purpose of this book is to explain how a variety of NLP techniques can be applied to change the way you think and act in your quest for losing weight and then staying slim for good. By working through the book you will first progressively remove or update any elements of your current mindset that prevent you from achieving your weight loss objectives. Next you'll be introduced to the NLP techniques that have been shown to make the biggest difference to those intending to lose weight. You will then be fully equipped with the right knowledge, skills and attitude, to implement the strategies that really work for you.

On occasions throughout this book I refer to NLP thinking, believing, knowing or saying. I appreciate that NLP is not a person and so can't think or say for itself, so where you read this it's just a shorthand way of referring to the practice of NLP or the thoughts and actions of NLP practitioners.

Keeping things simple

The purpose of *The NLP Diet* is very simple. Keep this in mind as you read the book. It will highlight the most common issues and challenges faced by anyone looking to lose weight and then illustrate a wide selection of techniques from the world of NLP that will help you to overcome these issues quickly and effectively. What you are trying to achieve is also very simple: you'd like to lose body fat and change your body shape. Do not make it more complicated than it needs to be.

If you feel yourself becoming stuck or overwhelmed with the task at hand, return to this notion. You're reading this book because currently you're not completely satisfied with the way you look and feel. You believe that it's possible to look and feel better than you do at the moment. To alter your current situation, all you need is an understanding of the specific changes you can make to this routine that will bring you different results. All you need to achieve this understanding is an open mind and a willingness to experiment.

For many people, losing weight is a full-time preoccupation with a range of barriers to success including lack of time, lack of motivation, lack of knowledge, lack of resources, slow results, no results, yo-yo results, cravings, feelings of being deprived, temptation, isolation, social pressure, unhappiness, confidence issues, frustration and negative self-image.

As with most things that matter in life, losing weight doesn't just happen by accident. You can't suddenly shed kilos just by thinking about it or because you want the right result more than ever this time. You need the right mindset for success supported by appropriate action and that's where NLP comes in. NLP is essentially a collection of techniques that can be used to 'reprogram' your brain in order to help you think differently, act differently, achieve new results and stay slim forever.

Does NLP work?

There are some people who are sceptical about NLP, sometimes because the techniques aren't fully grounded in science, sometimes because their only exposure to NLP has been through stage hypnosis, and sometimes simply because they've seen the techniques misused or applied inappropriately. My view is that if you like the idea of the techniques and you apply them to your situation and they work, then NLP is a successful intervention. If you feel that some techniques don't work for you, that's fine too. It may be that the timing isn't right and specific techniques will work for you in the future. In the meantime, there are plenty of others to try. What's important is that you're prepared to experiment and give these things a go. After all, if you're trying to lose weight, the only guaranteed way to delay your desired result is to do nothing at all.

Insight

The first step towards successful weight loss is to free yourself of any preconceptions about dieting and the results, positive or negative, that you associate with diets. For a moment set aside what may have happened in the past and allow yourself a new start with an open mind and no limitations on how you will go about achieving your goals.

A fresh approach

NLP believes that you cannot solve a problem with the same thinking that created the problem. This notion has never been more relevant than when it comes to losing weight.

It's likely that everyone you know has considered their weight at some point in their life. It's highly probable that the majority of people you know are either on a diet, have been on a diet or regularly consider what they eat and drink in relation to how it will affect their weight.

The difficulty many people have with losing weight is that they approach any new diet or new food routine with an outdated mindset. They know that what they've tried in the past didn't work, but they feel that by trying the same routine with renewed vigour, they may experience more positive results in the short-term. There always remains for most people, however, the nagging doubt that, because slipping backwards has followed positive results on a number of occasions in the past, the same process will repeat itself in the future. They begin their quest to lose weight thinking that some good results may be possible, but that they probably won't last that long. With this attitude you limit your potential results before you even begin.

The NLP Diet provides you with a new way to think about losing weight. An approach that is rooted in changing the way you think in order to guarantee quick and long lasting results. By thinking differently you will behave differently and, with this combination, you can be assured of achieving the results you have been looking for, sometimes for many years. And with this approach there are no backward steps: if you change the way you think now using these techniques, you change it forever. The approach is not a temporary quick fix that relies on you following a specifically prescribed routine, but a lasting, concrete, unshakable way of living life with a relationship with food and your weight that really works for you. Each chapter will help you piece together all the resources you require for lasting success with your weight management. By the end you will be in total control of your weight, your body shape, your eating habits and your energy levels.

Seeing is believing?

'Seeing is believing' is a phrase that many people are familiar with, and a concept that they experience on a daily basis. They see specific events and they believe this is how the world works. But let's examine the phrase a little more closely. Consider this for a moment. Just because something happens, does that event affect everyone who sees it in the same way? Do all participants in any given situation leave believing the exact same things took place?

NLP chooses to look at this phrase in reverse and suggests that, in actual fact, *believing is seeing*, and that what you believe is what you will see evidenced around you in the world. Your beliefs actually dictate what you see around you and these events then reaffirm your initial beliefs.

SO WHAT DO YOU BELIEVE WHEN IT COMES TO LOSING WEIGHT?

Your beliefs closely dictate your behaviour and your results in all areas of life but sometimes our beliefs can become outdated. So how do you uncover your beliefs around weight loss? Take a look at the following statements and assess which appear most familiar to you, which sound right to you or which sit most comfortably with you.

▶ Losing weight is easy.
▶ Losing weight is hard.
▶ I've struggled with my weight all my life.
▶ Losing weight shouldn't be difficult.
▶ Losing weight isn't the problem; it's my busy life that gets in the way.
▶ Diets work in the short-term.
▶ Losing weight is a good challenge.
▶ It's inevitable that you gain weight as you get older.
▶ Diets don't work.

Write out in a notebook all the thoughts that run through your head when you think about losing weight.

Now separate these thoughts, which are essentially your beliefs around losing weight, into two separate lists. The first list contains beliefs that will help you in your quest to lose weight; the second contains beliefs that are currently preventing you from achieving success with losing weight. Using a notebook, write out these two lists: entitle list one 'Thoughts in my head that help and support me in my quest to lose weight' and call list two 'Thoughts in my head that hinder me in my quest to lose weight'.

Every single thought that hinders you in your quest for weight loss is a limiting belief. Each time one of these thoughts enters your head it will slow any progress you are potentially able to make. These thoughts create conflict in your mind between what you want to achieve and what you think you are capable of achieving.

Limiting beliefs are not consciously created to make our lives more difficult but they can gradually form in our mind either because they were appropriate to our life at some point in the past, or they began as a way of justifying or excusing some type of behaviour.

For example, you may believe that losing weight is hard. This is a limiting belief that you may have decided to adopt because you have witnessed other people experience varying degrees of success or failure with different diets. Creating this belief served a purpose at the time it was formed; thinking that losing weight is hard spares you the time and effort of changing your behaviour in any way. But is this belief still relevant today? Is it helping you or hindering you in your quest to lose weight.

A new approach for new, improved results

This is a good time to make the distinction between this book, *The NLP Diet*, and other diets that you may have come across in the past. Most diet plans focus on the practicalities of dieting and losing weight, primarily, what you eat, when you eat it and how much you consume. They concentrate on changing your behaviour without paying too much attention to the thought processes that underlie why you are behaving in a way that's inconsistent with your weight management objectives in the first place.

The NLP Diet explores your past and current states of mind in order to refine your present attitudes and design those for the future that will be most beneficial to achieving your ideal weight loss and weight management strategies. With the correct mindset, essentially the 'why' you want to lose weight, devising the 'what' and 'when' of the healthy eating plan that works for you becomes quite straightforward.

You may believe that diets only work for the short-term because you have had some short-term success with diet plans in the past. You may believe that gaining weight as you grow older is inevitable because you have seen some people you know get heavier with the passing of the years. You may have good evidence for all of these beliefs but this doesn't mean they are true and absolute. Many people think diets do work because they have worked for them. In many cases, they simply have a different definition of 'diet' where they interpret the word in its original sense – what they eat and when they eat it – not as a specific food plan designed solely for losing weight, as determined by the latest experts and endorsed by any willing celebrities.

So think for a moment about your current situation. Do you believe in diets? Do you believe in healthy eating? Do you believe there's a solution out there for you?

Question your beliefs

There are a huge number of people who have discovered a food plan that doesn't only bring them short-term results but works for them for weeks and months and years.

Just because in the past you experienced only short-term success with a single plan or by selecting just a few of the many options for healthy eating doesn't mean this will be the result this time around.

For every person who gains weight as they get older, there will be someone who successfully maintains their weight year after year without giving it a second thought.

In many cases we select what we choose to see around us based on our beliefs, because we are unconsciously looking for reassurance that what we believe about the world is right. We like to think our ideas about the world are accurate because this makes things simpler than questioning and investigating everything we experience every day.

Often though, if you were to adopt a contrasting belief you would see just as much evidence to support it if you look carefully enough. To test this notion, try the following experiment. If you hold the belief that everyone gains weight as they get older, start looking out for anyone over the age of 40 who looks as though they're maintaining a consistent weight. You'll soon notice plenty of them. If you believe that losing weight is impossible within your busy schedule, seek out some people who've lost weight and find out how many of them have a quiet weekly routine with many spare hours to devote to their weight management. You might find them few and far between and instead come across a vast number of people creatively accommodating their weight loss into even the most chaotic routine.

LIMITING BELIEFS AND LIMITED WEIGHT LOSS RESULTS

You may by now have identified many limiting beliefs that you hold. Don't worry about this as the awareness of them is the first step in overcoming them. Specific limiting beliefs that lead to slow progress with weight loss feature on the list below. Add to this list with any that you feel are appropriate to you.

- ▶ I don't have any willpower.
- ▶ I'm too old to change now.
- ▶ I've got a sweet tooth.
- ▶ I'm greedy.
- ▶ I was meant to be fat.
- ▶ I have big bones.
- ▶ I have a heavy build.
- ▶ Everyone has their 'natural weight' and mine is just more than I'd like it to be.
- ▶ Healthy food doesn't taste of anything.
- ▶ Diets don't work.
- ▶ All my family is overweight so I don't stand a chance of being thin.
- ▶ Exercise is for crazy people.

A SUCCESSFUL BELIEF SYSTEM

Spring cleaning your belief system is like laying the ground work for making quick progress with weight loss. If you embark on another weight loss programme while maintaining the same beliefs, you'll experience the same results as you have in the past. To succeed efficiently you need to analyse your belief system and create a long list of current and up-to-date beliefs that will support you in your aims. Listed below are a few to get you started. Add as many of your own to this list as you like. You can come up with some new and

supportive beliefs simply by inverting current limiting beliefs.
This may not feel completely convincing right now, but with practice
and with the new evidence that you will now see all around you,
it soon will.

- ▶ Successful weight loss is merely a question of priorities.
- ▶ The results of losing weight are far more enjoyable than any
  potential distractions along the way.
- ▶ I am in charge of what I eat and drink.
- ▶ Everything I do is my choice.
- ▶ I live with the benefits of the choices I make with my food.
- ▶ Healthy eating gives me a buzz.
- ▶ Managing my weight makes me happy.
- ▶ Managing my weight gives me confidence.
- ▶ Taking responsibility for myself feels good.
- ▶ Healthy eating is forever.
- ▶ Diets don't work.

You'll notice the final successful belief is the same as the last item
on the list of limiting beliefs. This highlights a notion that NLP
touches on often, the notion of words, meaning and context being
all-important. To distinguish between these beliefs, the crucial factor
is context. If your belief that diets don't work stops you from
taking action, then you are clearly limiting your progress. If, on the
other hand, your belief that diets don't work leads to you quit
dieting and start eating healthily for successful weight management
for the long-term, you're in for a dramatically different result. So
don't just question the wording of your beliefs, take a closer look
at the sentiments behind them and the context in which you use the
words you choose. In many cases, the same words can be used for
dramatically different results.

As you analyse your core belief system you'll notice there are some
beliefs that are easy to change and others that are a little more deeply
rooted. You may resist questioning these for the moment, but don't
let this worry you. Often, the more deeply held and well established
the core belief is, the greater the potential victory when you are
finally able to investigate the reasons for this limiting belief and
then turn it into a belief that supports you.

To illustrate the power of updating your beliefs, here are a couple of
real life examples of belief change in action.

Sarah had a successful career that she loved. Until recently, her only complaint was that her busy work schedule made it impossible to eat healthily or take consistent exercise, with the result that since she began her working life she steadily gained weight year after year.

The belief that work prevented her from taking the time to eat well and exercise was a convenient notion for Sarah to cling onto back in the early days of her career, as it helped her avoid any feelings of guilt when she grabbed whatever food she could during a busy day, or skipped yet another exercise session. It soon became a limiting belief, however, as it repeatedly prevented Sarah from entertaining any new thoughts or strategies relating to how she was going to manage her weight effectively.

As time passed and taking control of her weight became more pressing, the first task for Sarah was to raise her awareness of this limiting belief, question it and come up with something more positive. The real breakthrough came when Sarah altered her mindset to not consider that losing weight, planning meals and taking exercise were all things that got in the way of her successful career, but rather to consider that these things were essential foundations to making her career even more successful in the future. Sarah's new belief system triggered a complete turnaround in her life resulting in new eating habits, a completely new exercise schedule and a weight loss of 11 kg (24 lb) over the course of seven months.

A simple two-step belief change
Old, core limiting belief: 'I'm too busy with work to do anything about losing weight.'

New, positive core belief: 'Eating well, taking exercise and losing weight are all fundamental to my ongoing success in business and do wonders for my confidence.'

The results of Sarah's simple belief change were dramatic. Here's what she had to say when asked how she was progressing.

Weight loss continues…I am very pleased to say I have dropped a dress size. I put an old suit on today and I couldn't wear the pants – they were too baggy. I have now lost 11 kg (24 lb) and have had to buy a new wardrobe!!! I feel great!

On average I am walking 10,000 steps per day (yesterday I did 17,000 just in the course of work). Am taking the stairs at work when I don't have heavy bags to carry and am now run/walking 4 km in 30 minutes, three times a week and it's having a very good effect on my tennis game and at netball. I have bought a Pilates band and DVD and am doing a session at home a couple of times per week and am really watching what I am eating (and drinking!)

I am receiving a lot of positive support from family and colleagues about the changes I have made and the changes they can see. I have more energy and am feeling really positive about work and life in general. The gym manager at work saw me in gym clothes coming out of the gym one day and was heard to say, 'Has hell frozen over?' She has been trying to get me into the work gym for about three years!!! Can I thank you sincerely for your encouragement to give new things a try. Do keep in touch – it's lovely to be able to give a positive account of how things are going.

Belief change in action 2: 'I can't run...can I?'

For years Ron had experienced a very successful career but was becoming increasingly distracted by thoughts of the toll his busy working life was taking on how he looked and how he felt. A short pause for thought and a little bit of planning one summer was enough to get Ron started on making some big changes.

The trigger to Ron's change of heart and the key to a new fitness and weight loss routine were actually quite simple. A few years ago Ron had injured himself running and decided this was due to the extra weight he had been carrying. At the time he had been around 20 kg (44 lb) overweight. From that moment onwards, to Ron's mind at least, his running days were over. Until that point, running had always been a regular feature of Ron's exercise and weight management routine and without it things began to slide.

Now, looking back on this period in his life, Ron chose to address his limiting belief that he was too old to run and instead replaced it

(Contd)

with a belief that running had been both enjoyable and a successful weight management technique in the past, so why shouldn't this be the case for the future as well. He wasn't injured any more so there was no longer any need for this to restrict him in his results.

A simple two-step belief change
Old, core limiting belief: 'I'm too old to run.'

New, positive core belief: 'There's absolutely no reason why running shouldn't be part of my regular weight management routine.'

I finished working with Ron in June and contacted him a month later to see how he was getting on. Subsequent, regular reports back from Ron on his progress over the following few months make interesting reading.

28 July: I'm very well. My action plan is going better than I thought. I continue to run almost every day. I'm maintaining a good food style: not only breakfast but also at lunch and dinner with little bread and a lot of vegetables. I'm trying to lose weight, and since the end of June I lost 2 kg (4.5 lb). I have stopped with coffee and my wellness feeling is getting better. I want to try to lose 5 kg (11 lb) before Christmas, to arrive to 85 kg (187 lb).

28 September: I'm glad to tell you I ran a half marathon in two hours! Just four months ago it sounded impossible: I lost more than 10 kg (22 lb) thanks to some simple changes to my food and my exercise routine.

10 May: I want to update the information about my performance. When I began the programme, my personal weight was 93 kg (205 lb) and now after ten and a half months, my weight is now 73 kg (161 lb). Last Saturday I ran my first marathon (before last May, running 5 km was a miracle) and I'm starting training for the New York Marathon in 2011. My work and personal life is totally different and I feel better, in particular regarding headaches and stomach-aches: I now only eat good food in the right quantities.

Insight
If you find it difficult to keep coming up with positive beliefs that support effective weight loss, ask other people who have been successful with losing weight and maintaining their target weight. Make a list as long as you can of all the options you have for beliefs that have worked for others and could work for you.

The right attitude

Your life so far has prepared you with everything you need to know to achieve your weight loss goals. You have the opportunity to ask whatever questions you need to help you design a selection of weight loss strategies. Have conviction that the changes you are making now will guarantee you success. Believe in your own abilities.

The right beliefs

Do not look to the world to reinforce beliefs that lead you away from weight loss success. Instead, analyse your current belief system, remove any limiting beliefs, and focus on beliefs that will support you on your journey to success.

10 THINGS TO REMEMBER

1 We begin forming beliefs at an early age and our belief system is refined over the course of our life.

2 Beliefs are formed for good reasons at the appropriate time.

3 Beliefs can be limiting or they can be liberating.

4 Your belief system can be updated at any time.

5 When you update your belief system you will see evidence to support your new belief all around you.

6 Updating your belief system opens up your mind to a world of new experiences and opportunities.

7 Changing your belief system can affect the company you keep.

8 Updating core beliefs will lead to dramatic results with your weight loss.

9 Review and revise your belief system on a regular basis.

10 You cannot solve a problem with the same thinking that created the problem.

2

Getting motivated

In this chapter you will learn:
- *how to motivate yourself away from weight management results you don't want*
- *how to motivate yourself towards weight management results you do want*
- *how setting SMARTER goals will work for you.*

You'll have noticed already that one of the fundamental elements of NLP is to question everything. Because it is accepted that 'if you keep on doing what you've always done, you'll always get what you've always got', the only way to change future results is to ask questions that uncover new information to help you develop in different ways.

Once you become accustomed to this way of thinking, you'll very soon fall into the habit of analysing all your regular thoughts, behaviours and actions in a new context. You'll begin to look beyond what is familiar, and ask yourself regularly why you do the things you do. It will become a natural process to put your behaviour under a microscope and ask yourself questions at a deeper and deeper level.

As you develop this skill, you'll also begin to engage in a different way with all the people that you come across as part of your daily routine, and you'll view every single situation that you find yourself in slightly differently. Some people have described the transition towards this way of thinking as creating a sense of 'active engagement' in your life, rather than feeling as though you are a passive observer. You become proactive rather than reactive. You take full responsibility for what happens to you rather than ever feeling like a victim of circumstances. For many, this transition marks the beginning of a new way of living and it is precisely this new way of analysing yourself, your behaviour and the wider world around you that will guarantee you new results.

This questioning process applies to all areas of your life and all time frames, including the past, the present and the future. Chapter 1 showed you how to question some of your beliefs that were formulated in the past, in order to recalibrate your belief system for the future. By doing this you can clearly see how outdated beliefs can inhibit future results, and how a simple review exercise can release you from limitations in this area. This is the first example in the book of NLP technique, which helps you to systematically become aware of, and then remove, barriers and limitations to your success.

Another key area where the techniques of deeper level questioning and preparing a clear path for future success prove valuable is when setting goals and objectives for your life.

There's a quote by Napoleon Hill, author of *Think and Grow Rich* that says, 'What the mind can conceive and believe, it can achieve.' NLP clearly supports this view that if you plan something in enough detail and with sufficient consideration and conviction, you'll be well on the road to making it a reality. We can see the application of this immediately when considering weight loss.

It's the thought that counts

Many people approach the task of weight loss with the mindset that they 'really need to lose weight' or they could 'really do with toning up a bit', or 'it would be nice to drop a few kilos'.

These initial thoughts are all very relevant but without subsequent action, they are just that, initial thoughts, and no more likely to become a reality than a passing thought that it would be good to get a better job, or how great it would be to be rich. The part of the process that makes the difference between a passing thought and this thought becoming a reality is the ability to take time to analyse the detail of these thoughts and work out, on every level, what would need to happen to bring them to life.

This means planning your future with as much clarity and in as much detail as you can possibly manage.

The secret to success when planning your future is to set aside time to decide specifically what you'd like to achieve and then create an initial strategy, including practical steps you can put into action immediately. You must then turn your strategy into action, observe the results you experience, review your strategy regularly and refine it based on practical experience. There is also one other crucial element involved in achieving any objective and that is the element of timing. This is particularly relevant when thinking about weight loss.

When is the right time for losing weight?

The intensity of the desire to lose weight will ebb and flow depending on your mood, the time of the day, particularly before, during and after mealtimes, the time of the year, your confidence levels, and the commitments you have to fulfil during each week. If you're having a good day at work and all is going well with the family, you might not give weight loss any consideration at all for a while. On the other hand, if you're feeling dejected and tired, you may become preoccupied with losing weight as the way in which all your problems can be solved.

What's my motivation?

Losing weight is a great example of an objective often formed using what's known as 'away from' motivation. The desire to shed kilos is triggered by wanting to move away from the current situation which is deemed to be undesirable, namely carrying extra body weight and looking and feeling a way that's not consistent with how you want to live your life. Developing motivation to move yourself away from any given situation can be very successful in quickly changing the way people behave, but it also has limitations.

With away from motivation you may be limiting the potential extent of your success because once you have moved away from the unacceptable situation you find yourself in, the motivation for further progress can wane and results will stall. Away from motivation can be short-lived in that, as soon as you achieve a degree of progress you feel relieved, lose your sense of urgency, and return to the behaviours that led you to the unacceptable situation in the first place.

Away from motivation can also be limited if it merely reinforces your resolve temporarily but doesn't actually lead to any behaviour change at all. Feeling fat in the morning can lead you to resolve to avoid wine that evening and cook a sensible meal but by the time you've got through a busy day, you feel that a glass of wine and some comfort food is just what you need to lift your mood. So, away from motivation can be very short-lived and can result in more thought than action.

Relying on away from motivation can be particularly treacherous when it comes to long-term weight loss. It works brilliantly if the sight of yourself in a dressing room mirror, or the tightness of a particular item of clothing gives you the incentive to change, but not so well if the changes you put in place to rectify the situation are planned only in the short-term. What happens in this situation is that you may change your pattern of eating or your exercise routine for just as long as it takes to move away from the situation you don't like but then return to your old ways as soon as you lose a few kilos. This leads you into a pattern of yo-yo weight loss and gain, which is very destabilizing for your metabolism and will usually result in short-term weight loss turning into a steady increase in weight over the medium- to long-term.

Worse still, as was the case with someone I once worked with, if you are spurred to action to move away from being too heavy and you change your behaviour, with the positive results that you lose weight and feel better and then celebrate your success with a boozy meal out, your results are never going to be any better than very short-term and potentially quite destructive in the long-term.

Here are some general examples of away from motivation relating to losing weight. These are the thoughts that jump into your head unbidden or the responses to daily experiences that give us a kick and let us know that something has to change.

▶ Your clothes feel too tight.
▶ You catch your reflection in the mirror and you don't like what you see.
▶ Feeling low energy repeatedly.
▶ Feeling low in confidence.
▶ You overhear a negative comment or observation on your shape from someone else.
▶ You suddenly feel that you can't continue living as you have been.

- You observe other people who you think are overweight and you suspect you may be on the way to becoming one of these people.
- A change in circumstances prompt the desire to look and feel better than you do now.
- It's 1 January and you don't want to feel the way you do at the moment for yet another year.

In your notebook, list all the personal examples you can think of, of 'away from' motivating factors. What thoughts and experiences would losing weight put an end to?

Using negative emotions to positive effect

As you sit and consider everything about the situation with your weight loss that you'd like to move away from, you may feel motivated to take action immediately. Chances are though that you might also feel a little bit flat. This can be a natural response when we take time to dwell on all the things about our self and our life that we're unhappy with. If this is the case, the most effective way to channel what you're feeling at the moment is to acknowledge what you're not happy with, and then quickly move onto how you will change this situation. Accept what you don't like and immediately begin planning what you would like to move *towards* instead.

Insight

Have you ever considered just how much time you spend each day allowing negative thoughts to flow through your head? Make it a habit from now on to check yourself and replace every negative thought with at least one positive thought. In time you'll begin to notice that you spend less time dwelling on negatives.

What are you aiming for?

Far more powerful than away from motivation is the idea of motivating yourself towards something desirable. You'll have experienced examples of towards motivation when you come across images in magazines, on television and in real-life encounters with someone who has the body shape you want. The thoughts that float through your head stimulated by these images or experiences may be fleeting, so it's a good idea to begin tuning in more carefully to ideas and experiences that you find motivating so that you can begin creating a future that contains these elements in as much detail as possible.

'Towards' motivation has the advantage over away from motivation in that it creates a situation where there are no limits to your success. As long as you can keep fuelling the fire of motivation with positive reinforcement of what you're aiming for, your results will keep coming, long after you've moved away from your original undesirable situation. Provided you pick your desired results carefully, and we'll explore how to do this in a moment, towards motivation is also more sustainable on a day-to-day basis. Rather than being linked to the mood of the moment, towards motivation remains consistent until you reach your chosen reality and beyond, if you keep updating specifically what you want out of your future.

Here are some examples of towards motivation. They are positive events or life experiences that provide compelling incentives to make progress with your weight loss objectives:

- ▶ getting married
- ▶ going on holiday
- ▶ attending a forthcoming social/family event
- ▶ a romantic date
- ▶ a forthcoming work event
- ▶ a new job
- ▶ a new you
- ▶ observing a role model living the life you would like to have.

Now make a list of things that you are motivated to move towards. What are the positive elements in your life that staying slim forever would achieve? What aspects of your life or your future do you perceive would be improved by losing weight?

Successfully motivating yourself towards something is easy. All it requires is a little time and planning and it is this planning time that makes all the difference between hoping for a great result and experiencing a great result. When you begin to spend time focusing on what you really want to move towards, you'll soon see that the speed and the resilience of your success is directly related to the degree of planning you are able to achieve.

Deepening your motivation

As you contemplate the factors that are motivating you to change, it's likely that you'll be able to isolate some elements of away from motivation and some elements of towards motivation. By exploring these factors in detail, you will be able to increase your motivation towards change and success. Copy the questions below, and write the answers in your notebook to help you with this process.

1 Facing up to reality:
    ▷ Where am I now with my weight management strategy?
    ▷ How near or far am I from what I think would be my ideal healthy eating routine for perfect weight management?

2 Exploring away from motivating triggers:
    ▷ If I continue as I am with my current weight management strategy, the results will be...
    ▷ If my current behaviour patterns around food become more extreme, the most negative consequences could be...

3 Exploring towards motivating triggers:
    ▷ The most important things I want to achieve with my weight management strategy are...
    ▷ If I can make positive changes to my weight management strategy, the biggest benefits will be...

How committed are you?

I'm sure your initial response to this question will be that you are utterly committed to losing weight but it's important to stop for a moment and consider how far reaching that commitment actually is. How does your current level of commitment compare to weight loss regimes of the past? Are you looking for the same results as in the past or different results? How might your current commitment level affect the results you are able to achieve, or how quickly you can achieve these results? The following questions will help you clarify your commitment level.

1 Are you planning for positive results, or just hoping something good will happen?

Regular passing thoughts that it would be good to lose weight indicate a vague desire for change, but without any further planning, nothing tangible will actually happen. Frequently expressing a desire, to yourself and to others, that you would like things to be different is not a solution to your situation. Desire is nothing without a clear plan and some concrete action.

2 Are you planning for limited results or taking action that will produce only limited results?

As soon as you move beyond passing thoughts about weight loss and start taking some action, you stand a much greater chance of experiencing some results. This moment usually occurs when people are in the away from motivation stage and they begin with small steps to make changes with what they eat and the activity they take. How long this period lasts is related to how committed they are to making changes for the long-term.

3 Have you set up a system for success?

Taking initial actions towards losing weight will generate some success but the speed and sustainability of these results is greatly enhanced when you take time to develop a formal strategy for success. This occurs when you make the transition from away from motivation and replace this with towards motivation. At this point you begin to plan your results in great detail. You can do this by devising your own approach to planning your future but there are one or two systems in common use that could help you speed up your progress. One system that many people are familiar with is setting SMART goals.

Insight

Your level of commitment to achieving any objective has a direct impact on your results. If you were to apply a simple rating system to your commitment, a score of one out of ten would lead to fairly limited results. Yes, you may be in a better position than your current one, but results may take a while and may not be enough to satisfy you. With a five out of ten commitment level your results will be far more dramatic. If you are able to rate your level of commitment at eight, nine, or even ten out of ten, you will be guaranteed an amazing result. Apply this commitment rating to all thoughts that run through your head relating to your weight loss and be honest about how committed you really are.

Get SMART, get slim

Setting SMART goals is one of the first steps in translating a desire into positive action. It is a great tool for investigating and bolstering your commitment level to any objective. SMART goals must be:

Specific
Measurable
Achievable
Realistic
Time framed

SPECIFIC

Rather than considering the vague notion of losing weight, you need to decide exactly how much weight you want to lose and then specify your first target weight. Instead of thinking it would be nice to lose a few kilos, put some details to your goal. Choose the weight you would like to be, and the date by which you'd like to reach that weight.

MEASURABLE

By knowing what you weigh now and what your target weight is, you will be able to measure your progress at every step of the way and you'll know exactly when you've reached your target. Without regular measurements, you won't have an accurate assessment of how you are progressing. This will make it difficult to know when you need to refine your approach and this can in turn hamper your progress.

ACHIEVABLE

It is not possible for most people to lose 20 kg (44 lb) in a single week so don't set yourself up for frustration by picking an impossible objective. The recommended rate of safe, healthy and sustainable fat loss is 1 kg (2 lb) per week so bear this in mind when thinking about your target weight.

REALISTIC

Don't look at your weight loss objective in isolation or as if it's the only thing you have going on in your life. If the only thing you have to think about on a daily basis is losing weight then you're in the fortunate position that you can formulate an ideal plan to help you reach your desired result. This is rarely the case however, and most people find themselves trying to fit their weight loss routine into an already busy schedule. If you are one of these people, you need to consider all your existing time commitments and how they will affect your progress with your chosen goal, then think consider carefully how much time, effort and energy you have to devote to losing weight. Only after you take your work, family, social and any other regular commitments into account can you realistically set your weight loss objectives.

TIME FRAMED

Setting vague and open-ended objectives, such as, 'I'm going to lose 5 kg (11 lb)' suggests that these objectives will be realized, but at what point in the future? These statements lack a sense of urgency and mean that there's always tomorrow to think about when you'll make a start. Strangely though, where objectives like this are concerned, tomorrow never comes. If you want to ensure success with your objectives, you need to plan the specific date by which they will be achieved and then review the progress you are making towards this deadline every single day.

The benefit of a clearly time-framed deadline is that it focuses the mind. You will have experience of situations where a fixed deadline has inspired you to great things. Sometimes we need deadlines to make progress with projects we don't enjoy or that we're not looking forward to. If deadlines work in situations like this, imagine how effective they could be when applied to objectives and projects that you are actually excited by.

A further reason why deadlines work well is that you know, very clearly at all stages, when you will have achieved your goal, and when you can enjoy the fruits of your labours. We often get motivated when we imagine how good it will feel to have achieved a particular objective. Imagine the extra motivation you'll be able to conjure up when you know the date by which you will experience these positive feelings.

Insight

Because it's likely that losing weight isn't the only thing on your agenda at the moment, it will be beneficial to run some of your other current priorities through the SMART goal process. This will help highlight where various objectives may conflict, and will ensure that you proceed with a balanced approach to making consistent progress with all your objectives and priorities and never feel that you have to compromise in any area of your life.

Beyond SMART goals

As always, the more detail you can add to any thought process, the greater your chances of success. With this in mind, you can build on SMART goals and create even SMARTER goals, the E being for exciting and the R for recordable.

EXCITING

If achieving your chosen goal isn't exciting to you then why bother chasing after it? If you're looking for new results in any area of your life, you need to change your behaviour, and changing behaviour requires effort. In order to make this effort, it's important that you are excited by your goals. Otherwise, any behaviour change will be limited or short-lived at best. Spend some time considering why you want to lose weight and why achieving the results you desire really matters to you. Highlight every aspect of your chosen goal that gets you excited.

If losing weight would just be 'a nice thing to have' in your life then, although you may make some progress, the results that you could achieve may be less dramatic than if you view losing weight as an absolutely essential part of your short-, medium- and long-term future, and you have explored in great detail why the prospect excites you and makes you feel motivated to action.

RECORDABLE

In order for you to make the best possible progress with your weight loss objectives, it's vital that you can write down what you'd like to achieve and keep track of your progress at every stage. You may think that it'll be enough to monitor what's going on in your head, but will you be able to keep all the details to mind when you are busy? Keeping records of what's going on means that you can be accurate about how things are progressing and you can make changes to your plans based on the results you see in front of you.

It doesn't only have to be a written record of what's going on. You can record measurements such as weight and body composition and plot these on a chart to quickly see things heading in the right direction, which can be very motivating. You can use photographs to chart your progress. This is a popular and very effective technique. You take a photograph of yourself each week standing in the same position, in the same clothes or even your underwear, and you will very clearly be able to see changes as the weeks progress. Some people, even those who take photographs in their underwear find it even more motivating to add some extra accountability by sharing the photographs with selected contacts on their preferred social networking site or blog.

Another method is record your progress on a simple tick list. Once you've decided on a plan that you think will get you to your chosen objective, you can draw up a schedule of behaviour and activities, stick it on the fridge and then put a tick by every day that you follow your chosen plan.

You can also keep audio records of your progress or a video diary if that's easier. Or you can use all of these techniques, as the combination will really help to focus all your senses on what you're doing. Words, photographs and video make it easy to see how you are progressing and an audio or video record will help you clarify your thoughts as you develop your ongoing plan.

NLP tools to help you stay slim for good

▶ **Towards motivation**
   Focus on the positive results you want, not the negative consequences you don't want.
▶ **Deep and lasting motivation**
   Add layers of detail to your desired objectives to the point where your motivation to achieve them is unshakeable.
▶ **SMART & SMARTER goals**
   Spend time examining your objectives from all angles.

10 THINGS TO REMEMBER

1 Learn to question everything you do.

2 Practise becoming more engaged with the world around you.

3 Think of staying slim forever as a top priority, not just something that you should or ought to address.

4 Analyse all 'away from' motivating factors affecting your weight management.

5 Analyse all 'towards' motivating factors affecting your weight management.

6 Top up your towards motivation every day.

7 Be honest with yourself about the long-term implications of your current behavior.

8 Take time to consider what will motivate you to adopt new ways of behaving.

9 Plan the details of your future success.

10 Your current approach should include greater time and consideration than previous attempts at weight management. This is the key factor in getting a different result this time.

3

Planning for complete success

In this chapter you will learn:
- *how to plan the finer details of your chosen weight management results*
- *about visualizing your future to fast-track your results*
- *a step-by-step process to removing all barriers to quick and lasting weight loss.*

Goal setting with NLP

SMART and SMARTER goals have proved successful for many people, so NLP has devised a way to move beyond both of these systems and has come up with the idea of well-formed outcomes. To develop well-formed outcomes is to analyse and assess your desired results at a much deeper level than you would when working with any other system.

Insight

This process looks quite involved at first glance but don't let this put you off. First, be reassured that the process of analysing your chosen objective in this much detail will ensure more positive results than you've achieved in the past. Second, as you practise the technique, you'll find that these questions automatically crop up in your mind as you are considering future plans and goals. In reality, the process is never as formal as it appears here and you will become accustomed to continually making unconscious assessments based on the list of questions.

The key parts of the process of designing well-formed outcomes are as follows. Read through the headline questions first to familiarize yourself with them and then we'll look at each element in turn. When you follow the detailed explanation, it's a good idea to make some notes on how these statements help to focus your thoughts specifically on what you'd like to achieve with your weight loss.

- State your outcome as a positive experience.
- Establish precisely where you are now in relation to your outcome.
- Ask yourself, 'What will I see, hear and feel when I achieve my outcome?'
- Establish how you will know when you have achieved your outcome.
- Ask yourself, 'What will achieving this outcome do for me?'
- Check that your chosen outcome is created by you and will benefit you.
- Establish what resources you will need to achieve your outcome.
- Calculate and be aware of any costs or consequences to you or anyone else of you achieving your outcome.
- Make sure your chosen outcome is within your control.
- Check that your objective is truly exciting, compelling and desirable.
- Finally, be clear on your first action.

So, how does an understanding of well-formed outcomes help you lose weight? Follow the process and add as much information that's relevant to your personal situation as you can at each stage.

WELL-FORMED OUTCOMES: STEP 1

State your outcome as a positive experience.

For example, 'Today I'm embarking on a healthy eating routine that will ensure I achieve my ideal body and am then able to maintain this. My desired result is that I weigh 70 kg (154 lb) and my interim body weight targets will reduce at a rate of 0.5 kg (1 lb) a week for the next 14 weeks until I reach my ideal weight.'

WELL-FORMED OUTCOMES: STEP 2

Establish precisely where you are now in relation to your outcome.

The more details you can gather around where you are now in relation to your chosen outcome and how things will be different in the future, the better. As far as a diet or healthy eating plan is concerned, it's useful not simply to focus on weighing yourself, as scales can sometimes be deceptive. It's important to your long-term progress that you remain motivated at all times, so in addition to tracking your weight, measure your current body fat percentage and identify a variety of items of clothing that you can use to track your progress.

Write down what you'd like your body fat percentage to be at specific points in the future and line up the clothes that might not feel completely comfortable right now but that you will enjoy wearing in the future when you've changed your body shape. It's a great idea to have a selection of outfits that you feel you'll be able to get into at a variety of points in the future – a pair of trousers you'd like to get into in three to four weeks, a dress you'll be comfortable wearing in seven to eight weeks and so on.

Write down what you think the ideal food routine that will guarantee you reach your objectives will look like. Then establish exactly what's going on with your food routine at the moment. The best way to make sure you gather a true representation of what you eat and drink is to keep a food diary for at least a week. For best results in the future, the food diary should be honest and accurate and should begin immediately. Don't wait to begin your diary based on the fact that this week isn't a typical week. For most people there is no typical week and when it comes to healthy eating, one of the ways to ensure optimum results is to devise strategies for meals and snacks that stand up to *all* circumstances. It's easy to eat well when things are calm and quiet, the real challenge can be staying on track when things are busy.

WELL-FORMED OUTCOMES: STEP 3

Ask yourself, 'what will I see, hear and feel when I achieve my outcome?'

NLP is keen that we use all our senses to increase our ability to communicate and succeed in life. This includes sight, sound, touch, taste and smell. Tapping into all these senses enables you to create crystal clear images in your mind of how things will be once your outcome is made real. The reason this is important, as Napoleon Hill said, is that as soon as you begin imagining success, the closer you are to achieving it in reality. A powerful example of how this principle works in practice, relating to weight loss, is the idea of a forthcoming wedding.

Understandably, everyone wants to look their best on their wedding day, and for many people that means dropping a few kilos. You probably know a few people who have managed to get great results with their weight loss prior to their wedding, even when they may have struggled to get the same results with previous attempts in the past. So what makes the difference? Did those people employ some dramatically different behaviour or did they simply approach the challenge with a different mindset? Chances are they simply applied some knowledge they already possessed, and had probably made use of in the past, but because there was a stronger element of motivation surrounding their objective this time, and a clear emphasis on 'towards' motivation, the results were much improved.

The anticipation of the big day allows people to visualize very clearly how they want to look and what they want to see on the faces of others when the guests look at them. In their head they can already clearly hear other people saying how spectacular they look, and they imagine their guests commenting among themselves on how they managed to lose so much weight and get in such good shape. They also begin imagining what it will feel like to slip into a dress or a suit in exactly the size they want and they can already anticipate the rush of happiness this will give them.

They imagine the tastes and smells at every stage of the event, and everything is just that little bit sweeter, sharper and more intense because they are oozing with confidence and satisfaction in what they have achieved. Because most weddings require a lot of preparation, these positive thoughts run through the bride or groom's head many times a day for a period of months, continually reinforcing desire to make these thoughts a reality and underlining the importance of behaving in accordance with achieving their chosen outcome, so much so that they very rarely wander off track, and if they do, they very quickly recover their focus.

Take time now to think about what you will see, hear, feel, taste and smell when your weight loss outcome becomes reality and make time during every day from now on to consolidate these thoughts. Continue the list below, in your own notebook, with all the sights and sounds associated with your weight loss success. Revisit this list and add to it as often as you can.

- ▶ What will I see, hear and feel when I achieve my outcome?
- ▶ Friends report back that they and other people have noticed how good I look.
- ▶ I enjoy what I see when I look in the mirror.
- ▶ I feel a sense of satisfaction when shopping for, and wearing, new clothes.
- ▶ I experience a new sense of confidence.

▶ My family compliment me on how I look and what I have achieved.

▶ I see myself out having a good time. I picture these events both through my own eyes and also through the eyes of others observing the new me in action.

WELL-FORMED OUTCOMES: STEP 4

Establish how you will know when you have achieved your outcome.

With any objective, it's important to be clear on what constitutes success. For losing weight, you can measure the obvious indicators already mentioned such as your weight and body fat percentage. Remember also to look out some specific items of clothing that you know you can only wear comfortably when you are at your ideal weight and body shape.

It's likely that you will also be in possession of a new frame of mind when you achieve your outcome and it helps to be clear on what this will be right from the outset.

For example, you might know you've achieved your outcome when you look in the mirror and experience a feeling of satisfaction, rather than a sense of dejection. You might know you've been successful when you feel confident as you go about your daily routine rather than feeling self-conscious. You might imagine yourself shopping for clothes more often or with a different attitude when you do. It's likely that you'll be wearing different clothes or feeling very different in some of the clothes that you wear currently. You may envisage yourself socializing more or making changes in your life that you've previously shied away from.

Write down in your notebook all the ways in which you will know when you have achieved your outcome. This list should include the thoughts and feelings that you will be experiencing when you have achieved your outcome, as well as all the different ways in which you'll be behaving in the future.

WELL-FORMED OUTCOMES: STEP 5

What will achieving this outcome do for me?

It's important to understand exactly why you want this objective to become a reality. Losing weight may allow you to fit into different clothes and help you to feel more comfortable in many of the outfits you wear currently, but what else will becoming slimmer do for you?

Will it help you achieve a sense of satisfaction? Will it boost your confidence? Will it help you get a better job? Will it help you find a partner or improve your relationship with the partner you already have? It might, but these results aren't guaranteed.

To help you establish exactly what achieving your outcome will do for you, first, get clear on the *guaranteed* results you will experience by losing weight. Results such as decreasing your body fat percentage, changing shape and fitting into smaller clothes. Secondly, write out all the *possible* results you *may* experience. Having an idea of all possible results you could achieve makes it easier to review your progress against these anticipated results on a regular basis.

It may be that some of the results you anticipated from slimming down fail to materialize, or you discover they actually require an additional strategic approach. For example, you may have an idea that losing weight will improve your confidence levels and help you find a relationship. While this could happen, it's important to be clear that the three outcomes are not inextricably linked. It is possible to lose weight, gain confidence and find a relationship but there's no guarantee of this sequence of events.

This is why regular review of your progress against *all* your desired outcomes is crucial. If you think one outcome is directly linked to another you may end up feeling slightly disappointed, despite making great progress with one or even two of your desired results. By reviewing the correlation between your success with weight loss and your increased confidence, in relation to your ability to find a partner for example, you may decide there are other elements to the third part of your envisaged future life and that new and different strategies are required to complete the picture.

It's likely that achieving success with your initial desired outcome of losing weight will put you in a better position to tackle many other goals that you would like to achieve in life. What we're saying here is that to improve your ongoing success with everything you tackle in your life, be very clear at all stages which actions and which plans are related to which outcomes and make sure your daily behaviour reflects your priorities for success in all areas.

To help with establishing specifically what achieving your weight loss goal will do for you, complete the following list in your notebook, including details of everything that success with weight loss will

directly enable you to do, as well as secondary benefits that success
with weight loss will pave the way for in due course.

- ▶ What will achieving this outcome do for me?
- ▶ What are the guaranteed results of my losing weight?
- ▶ What might be the secondary results associated with my losing
  weight?

WELL-FORMED OUTCOMES: STEP 6

**Check that your chosen outcome is created by you and will
benefit you.**

There's no better way to hamper your chances of weight loss success
than to take on the project because someone else suggested it, or
because you suspected someone else thinks it's the right thing for you
to do. Any challenge you take on can quickly lose momentum when
it comes to staying motivated, if it was someone else's idea. For quick
success, you need ownership of a project and total responsibility for
what happens along the way.

Think of a time when someone else suggested that you take on
a challenge, event or project. It may have been a diet, or it could
have been the idea of a promotion at work, a sporting challenge, or
attending a social engagement. It could even be as simple as following
someone's advice on what to wear or even what to choose for lunch?
Think about how each of these events turned out.

The drawback when we're acting on the advice of others is that often
we encounter a little bit of internal resistance. Fundamentally, we
know what's best for us and if the suggestions of others go against
our own instincts of what's right at the time, even in the smallest
degree, the resistance you experience to following this path can
seriously affect your possible results.

Now think of a time when you made an important choice or decision
in life. Remember when a light bulb suddenly came on, something
just clicked and you felt you knew how you wanted to progress in
a situation. You may have done plenty of research and gathered
opinions from a number of trusted people but ultimately the decision
was yours. When this happens – when you experience a breakthrough
moment and the timing is right for what you decide to embark upon –
your ability to perform can be incredible. These are the moments
when you feel very focused and you're fully convinced that what

you're doing is right for you. You are suddenly able to make progress where you may have struggled in the past, and you see opportunities to succeed where before you may have seen obstacles.

When you decide that you want something in your life, your mind begins stacking positive reasons to make these things happen and these thoughts fuel your motivation every single day. This motivation leads to positive action which in turn leads to positive results which leads back to even greater motivation. There's very little more motivating than a taste of success and when you feel you're making progress sparked by your own desires and efforts, you will be quickly galvanized towards further motivation and action.

WELL-FORMED OUTCOMES: STEP 7

Establish what resources you will need to achieve your outcome.

Everything you require to achieve success with weight loss is within your control. Either you have the knowledge that will lead you to the result you're looking for, or you have access to the resources that will provide you with the answers. You are embarking on a project that many other people have researched and studied and millions have had success with. So you needn't be particularly concerned about the 'how' of successful weight loss. All the information you require exists already and with the right attitude and incentives, you will find access to everything you need. Your key to success is to thoroughly clarify the 'why' attached to your weight loss objectives, which is what you are doing as you work through the process of creating a well-formed outcome.

To focus your mind on the resources you need, make a list of everything you require for the journey to success. Title this list 'Resources I need in place to achieve my chosen outcomes'. Things like a pair of trainers to exercise in, access to research on ideas for different meals and snacks, a support network, a selection of challenges to keep you on track, child care while you shop for and prepare some of the food you need for your healthy eating plan. All the knowledge you will require for successful weight loss is out there in the form of books, CDs, DVDs, websites and forums. There are countless products in shops and online. One of the key resources you'll require is time and for this you need to have your support network in place, good planning skills and a willingness to do things slightly differently from the ways in which you've done them in the past.

Good preparation is vital here and if you lay the foundations for the specific resources you need access to on a day-to-day basis, you'll be amazed at how inventive you can be to make sure that everything you need is in place when you need it.

WELL-FORMED OUTCOMES: STEP 8

Be aware of any costs or consequences to you, or anyone else, of you achieving your outcome.

To ensure success, you need to approach your desired outcome without hesitation or reservation. This means making sure that no aspect of your life will change for the worse when you reach your goal. For weight loss, any anticipated costs are usually perceived to be things such as missing out on treats such as food items or drinks that we feel make up our weekly routine and without which, life just wouldn't be the same.

If you find yourself in this situation, the easiest solution is to decide what level of consumption of these items is acceptable for the future. You need to make sure that you don't feel you're missing out, but instead that it will be possible to include the items you fear would be a loss to your routine, provided you eat them in the right amounts and at the right times. An ongoing food diary will help you establish how much and how often is appropriate for food 'treats' or 'vices' such as chocolate, cakes, pastries, sweet drinks and alcohol.

Consider also how your family and friends will react to the new you. It's likely that the physical changes that take place with your weight loss will affect you mentally and, if they do, how will you cope with this and how will others cope? Is there a chance that your relationship with any of the people you are close to will change? If so, how do you anticipate your relationships changing, and which relationships are most likely to change? If you are able to anticipate any likely costs or consequences of you achieving your outcome, you can use this information to refine your approach and your attitudes and how you choose to interact with everyone around you regularly along the way. This regular updating of your communications and interactions will minimize the likelihood of any dramatic differences of opinion arising in the future. By giving everyone a chance to become gradually accustomed to the new you, there are no shocks further down the line.

NLP suggests four specific questions that will help you explore the costs and consequences of your behaviour for you and those around you. Answer these questions in as much detail as possible allowing yourself time to consider the questions in relation to as many different areas of your life and as many of your relationships as possible. List all the thoughts that come to mind.

▶ What will happen if you achieve this outcome?
▶ What won't happen if you achieve this outcome?
▶ What will happen if you don't achieve this outcome?
▶ What won't happen if you don't achieve this outcome?

WELL-FORMED OUTCOMES: STEP 9

Make sure your chosen outcome is within your control.

I'm sure you're familiar with the feelings of stress and frustration. Most people experience them at some stage. These feelings arise when we sense something in our life is out of control.

If you're trying to lose weight, you may feel circumstances drifting out of your control at work, for example, if you need to eat out to entertain clients, if your office canteen has limited healthy options or you are unable to have access to the meals or snacks that you've prepared during long meetings. At home you may feel frustrated if you find it difficult to cook and eat what you'd like or monitor your food intake or portion sizes with family members around you distracting you.

Stress is the enemy of effective weight loss, so the first thing to do is not to give in if you feel circumstances are drifting beyond your control. For every situation that arises, simply pause and take stock first of what elements of the current situation you *can* take control of – and there will always be some – and second, focus on how you can prevent the same situation happening again in the future. This immediately puts you back in charge of your long-term weight loss destiny.

A change in mindset can also be helpful here and this involves seeing every possible frustration as an opportunity. Frustrations can arise when everyday life gets in the way of what you are trying to achieve. But everyday life is just that: the tests and challenges that you actually have to navigate around in your quest for success. So instead of becoming frustrated, get specific about what you do to avoid these situations or deal with them more effectively in the future. There will be challenges along the way; it's how you deal with them that matters.

Stress can be a barrier to success with any outcome, but it is a particularly important consideration when it comes to losing weight. The reason is that too much stress, or even a small amount of stress on a consistent basis, can have a detrimental effect on how your body fuels itself, particularly with regard to burning body fat. In an environment with regular stress, the body can become too reliant on fuelling itself with adrenalin and sugar and may actually become ineffective at burning calories from fat sources. If this situation persists for too long, it can be difficult to reverse. Stress also makes your body less able to digest and process the food that you consume, so even a healthy diet may not be as effective as it could be when introduced into a stressed system. Finally, stress can create an environment where your exercise becomes less effective at fat burning because your body is just too used to relying on adrenalin.

Insight

Making sure that your weight loss goal is within your control is probably one of the most important keys to success. Remaining in control of your objectives comes down to managing your expectations of how each day and each week is going to pan out. Take charge and make meticulous plans, but be flexible with your plans and spend a little time each day updating and reviewing them. By remaining flexible you will always feel in control of your weight loss. If you lose this feeling of being in control, you risk a temporary pause or a complete halt in your progress. It's worth mentioning at this point that one of NLP's presuppositions – one of the core ideas of NLP – encapsulates exactly this idea. It says, 'in any system, the person with the most flexibility will control the system'. In this case, the 'system' is made up of anything and anyone involved with your quest to lose weight. You will remain in control of the system if you are able to take charge of all circumstances you find yourself in.

WELL-FORMED OUTCOMES: STEP 10

Check that your objective is truly exciting, compelling and desirable.

Does the thought of losing weight excite you? There's a big difference between something that would be 'nice to have' in life, an added bonus to your daily routine, and something that is a 'must have'. Think of a time when you really wanted something in your life. Remember how the desire to reach the end result got you fired up and kicked into action. Remember the feeling of achievement when you finally reached success.

You can also think about times when you thought you wanted something but it wasn't a desperate priority. Were you able to make that desire a reality?

If you're going to make changes in your life, you need to get fired up about what these changes will lead to. You must think about succeeding with your objective and use these thoughts to create circumstances where you are as excited at the prospect of getting started as you are by the prospect of your ultimate success.

As well as the initial idea of what you would like to achieve being exciting, working to the appropriate time frame is also crucial. Even the most exciting goal can lose its appeal if the idea of success is too far in the future.

I once worked with someone who set an objective of losing 3.5 kg (8 lb) in 18 months. While a goal like this is specific and time framed, it's lacking any sense of urgency or excitement and is unlikely to lead to immediate action. In fact this person could have waited for 16 or even 17 months before getting started and still achieve their chosen result. Setting objectives that aren't challenging enough is as bad as picking a challenge that isn't realistic.

Write down why reaching your target weight and staying slim for good is truly exciting, compelling and desirable for you.

WELL-FORMED OUTCOMES: STEP 11

Be clear on your first action.

Planning is crucial and action is vital. Immediate action is even better. Once you've explored your outcome in as much detail as possible, you must be clear on what immediate actions are required to set you on the right track. Actions could be grabbing a healthy snack, compiling a healthy shopping list, looking up some new recipes or taking some exercise. Whatever you choose, do it as soon as possible.

Taking immediate action is a very clear message to your brain that you are now on the road to achieving your outcome, rather than still waiting to get started. This change in attitude instantly overcomes the issue of frustration attached to the feeling that you really want to get started soon but things keep arising that get in your way. Each action that you take brings with it a sense of control and confidence that steadily grows and provides motivation to continue in the same vein. These actions accumulate and gradually reinforce your internal thought processes that you are responsible for the way you behave and that you can be successful in doing what you know is right.

NLP tools to help you stay slim for good

Well-formed outcomes

Quiz yourself thoroughly to about your plans for the future in order to create the perfect environment for guaranteed results. The more detail you can add to your plans, the more likely they are to become a reality.

10 THINGS TO REMEMBER

1 Success with any goal requires an approach that is different from the approaches of the past.

2 The more detail you can create in your head around success with your objective, the easier your goals will be to realize.

3 Be specific about when you want to achieve success.

4 Systematically remove all obstacles to success, be they real or imagined.

5 Visualize success every day until you experience it.

6 Take your first action towards your goal as soon as possible.

7 Take consistent action towards your goal every single day.

8 As you work on your chosen objective every day, you should feel excited about your progress and the end result.

9 If your objective loses its sparkle for you, analyse what elements of it you need to revise in order to rekindle the urgency around making it happen.

10 Stay in control of your objective at all times.

4

Your future on your terms

In this chapter you will learn:
- *how to maintain balance in your life while achieving your weight management goals*
- *how to plan for short-, medium- and long-term results*
- *how to channel the power of your unconscious mind to help you lose weight.*

Outcome planning and a sense of purpose

Gaining clarity on what you'd like to achieve in any area of your life is a great asset in your ability to turn planned outcomes into reality. Something to bear in mind at all times is that it's unlikely that you will ever have only one objective to focus on. If you did, life would be simple. Imagine embarking on your plan to lose weight with no other commitments on your schedule. Your journey could be so easy.

Because your life is full of many different elements, it's useful to examine them all together rather than in isolation. This helps clarify just how many things you're trying to achieve at any given time. It's also helpful to consider the objectives you have that span different time frames so that you don't become too fixated on one particular period of your life. There are a number of reasons this strategy works.

Life is about balance and you will ultimately feel more fulfilled if you can make progress with a number of projects at the same time. It's also important to make sure that victory in any given area of life does not come at the cost of progress in other areas. To achieve this you must stay in control of all areas of your life. It's also more likely that you will stay on track in any given area if you can see clearly how success in one area impacts positively on other aspects of your life.

For example, an objective of eating healthily and losing weight is more likely to become a reality if you can clearly see eating healthily within the context of other areas of your life, such as increasing energy to fulfil work demands that will lead you to the promotion you want, or simply make you more efficient and able to leave the office earlier. Alternatively you might see success with healthy eating as a way to keep your mood positive so that you can be at your best, mentally and physically, to fulfil your family obligations. Or you may view success with losing weight as the most likely route to boosting your day-to-day confidence.

When I first came across NLP, one of the tools that I found most useful was a planning framework that enables you to look at your priorities for a number of different areas of life over a selection of time frames. I've used this tool with clients ever since as it is a very effective way of highlighting a number of priorities and then scheduling them effectively so they all complement each other and become more likely to work successfully in combination, rather than any outcomes causing problems with regard to time or resources required for other outcomes. Another reason that a comprehensive outcome planner is so valuable is that when you set to work creating one for yourself and then use it to begin achieving positive results, you will quickly be able to identify the strategies that help you to succeed in one area and you can then apply these strategies elsewhere.

Planning the results you want and when you want them

A detailed outcome planner is a way to put your weight management objectives in perspective and add variety, depth and momentum to your reasons for making them work for you. Losing weight for the sake of losing weight is one thing. Losing weight as an integral part of progressing your life in a number of ways provides you with many compelling reasons to stay on plan and, as you know, the more good reasons you have to make your plan a reality, the less likely you are to wander off track at any stage.

	1 month	2 months	3 months	4 months	5 months	6 months
Health, wellbeing & weight loss	2 × weekly gym visits; 1 × long walk; target weight: 69 kg (152 lb); experience increased energy	2 × weekly gym visits; 1 × long walk; target weight: 67 kg (148 lb); experience increased energy	2 × weekly gym visits; 1 × long walk; 1 × swim; target weight: 65 kg (143 lb); experience increased energy	2 × weekly gym visits; 1 × running; 1 × swim; target weight: 63 kg (139 lb)	1 × weekly gym visit; 1 × running; 1 × swim; sign up for a team sport; target weight: 62 kg (136 lb)	1 × weekly gym visit; 1 × running; 1 × swim; 1 × weekly team practice; target weight: 60 kg (132 lb)
Intimate relationship	Plan quality time with my partner	Refine the routine that works best for both of us	Maintain the routine that works best for both of us	Maintain the routine that works best for both of us	Review the routine that works best for both of us	Maintain the routine that works best for both of us
Family	Devise a schedule for some quality family time	Include family members in my activity routine, i.e. family walks	Include family members in my healthy eating routine	Maintain optimum health for all the family	Maintain optimum health for all the family	Maintain optimum health for all the family
Work	Devise a plan for increased efficiency at work	Devise a plan for more delegation at work	Create a plan for career development	Keep my plan for career development in mind at all times	Keep my plan for career development in mind at all times	Begin process of promotion or finding a new job

	1 month	2 months	3 months	4 months	5 months	6 months
Finances	Make a plan for effective spending	Consider options to boost my income	Act on options to boost income	Act on options to boost income	Income boosted by 10 per cent	Maintain increased income
Personal development	Research further study	Research further study; develop a more positive attitude	Sign up for further study	Begin further study; maintain my positive attitude	Maintain study routine	Maintain study routine
Social	Arrange walks with a friend; plan one night out a week	Investigate social events at the gym	Arrange swimming with a friend	Extend socializing with gym contacts; meet new people through study; design a routine to keep up with other friends as well	Meet new people at team sport; plan 1–2 nights out a week	Maintain a good balance with socializing
Hobbies	Explore options for a new hobby	Experiment with new hobby ideas	Experiment with new hobby ideas	Maintain new hobby/ies	Maintain new hobby/ies	Maintain new hobby/ies

WHAT GOOD LOOKS LIKE: PLANNING FOR RESULTS

The above table is an example of how your planner could look to begin with. The headings on the left are suggestions and you can substitute them for anything more appropriate to your routine if you feel you have other or additional life areas you'd like to include.

Think about how a plan such as the one above can change how you feel about losing weight. Very quickly you stop thinking about weight loss as just another thing on your to do list, and start thinking about it as just one aspect of many interesting challenges you have on your agenda. Losing weight will quickly develop from being an isolated objective to becoming a crucial element of your life that underpins success in many other areas. In this example, weight management objectives go hand in hand with greater confidence, more energy, a better social life and more fulfilling work and leisure time.

Planning in this way also helps you to see clearly how things will progress steadily over time. You know when you'll have succeeded with various objectives and this can take the pressure off the desire to achieve everything right now and mean that you take a more measured, progressive approach.

CREATING YOUR LONG-TERM FUTURE

Once you've put together a plan that will see you through the next six months, you can extend your planning further into the future. It may feel as though there are a few more grey areas as you plan this far ahead, but remember this document is a guide that can be regularly revisited and updated as necessary. What matters most is that you give some thought to the future you're going to be living. Here's an example.

	9 months	12 months	18 months	2 years	5 years
Health, well-being & weight loss	Maintain exercise routine and target weight	Set some exercise/ activity objective; group challenge or charity event	Review exercise routine and add any new components necessary to keep interest	Set some exercise/ activity objective; group challenge or charity event	Review exercise routine and add any new components necessary to keep interest
Intimate relationship	Continue quality time with my partner	Plan specific events together to deepen relationship	Continue regular reviews of relationship and associated actions	Continue regular reviews of relationship and associated actions	Continue regular reviews of relationship and associated actions
Family	Regular family meetings to bring everyone up to date with current priorities	Review family routine in light of education/ development/ enjoyment for all	Review family routine in light of education/ development/ enjoyment for all	Review family routine in light of education/ development/ enjoyment for all	Review family routine in light of education/ development/ enjoyment for all

(Contd)

	9 months	12 months	18 months	2 years	5 years
Work	Interviews complete for new position	New position under way	Keep my plan for career development in mind at all times	Look around for new job options	Keep my plan for career development in mind at all times
Finances	Continue ventures to boost income	New position brings increased salary	Continue ventures to boost income	New position will increase salary	Continue ventures to boost income
Personal development	Maintain study routine	Maintain study routine; look for new study challenges	Maintain study routine; look for new study challenges	Maintain study routine; look for new study challenges	Maintain study routine; look for new study challenges
Social	Maintain a good balance with socializing	Maintain a good balance with socializing	Maintain a good balance with socializing	Maintain a good balance with socializing	Maintain a good balance with socializing
Hobbies	Consider new hobbies to take me out of my comfort zone	Experiment with new hobbies to take me out of my comfort zone	Continue new hobbies that take me out of my comfort zone	Review hobbies	Review hobbies

Outcome planning and the unconscious mind

A detailed outcome planner also helps you to fully engage and make use of the power of your unconscious mind. The power of the conscious mind is an amazing thing. We can all use it to plan, communicate, solve problems and point our lives in any direction we wish. The unconscious mind is like the 'back office' of your brain. It's where much of the maintenance work of life takes place, as well as being the place where some of the most crucial decisions are worked through.

The unconscious mind is like our very own autopilot system, allowing us to perform many tasks without dedicating too many conscious resources to them. Driving is a great example of this. For the majority of the time spent driving, you don't give much conscious thought to either the process of keeping the car moving, stopping it when necessary or responding to the road and conditions around you. Only when something out of the ordinary occurs does the unconscious mind encourage you to engage your conscious mind and take the necessary action.

In many cases the unconscious mind is actually more effective than the conscious mind and instinctive reactions can feel more natural than when you try to think too much about how to react. The next time you're driving, and conditions are safe, try to think about every move you make and you'll find that it actually makes driving more difficult. As soon as you start to engage with the speed of the car, the movement of your feet to brake and work the clutch and the movements of your hands to steer and change gear, it feels as though there is too much to think about. It's like being a learner driver all over again.

Your unconscious mind is brilliant at problem solving, if you give it the chance. You'll know this if you've ever wrestled with a problem until you could see no way out of it only to have the solution present itself to you as soon as you move onto something else. In this situation you simply need to give your conscious mind a break and allow your unconscious mind an opportunity to work on the problem. It's similar when you wake up in the morning with the solution to a situation you couldn't get clarity on the previous day. While you sleep, your unconscious mind has an opportunity to process and organize your thoughts, make sense of the day's events and present solutions that had not previously occurred to you.

The great thing is that you can learn to use your unconscious mind to your advantage. You can give it information to process and ask it to provide you with solutions. You can also fine tune it to help you through your daily routine. By planning how you would like your days, weeks, months and years to run, and what results you are looking for out of life, you can equip your unconscious mind to filter information, spot opportunities and dictate actions and behaviours that will help you fulfil your objectives. This is why it is so important to make conscious decisions on what you'd like your future to look like and also important to regularly update your plans – to ensure that your unconscious mind is working on current, relevant and top priority objectives. Draw up your own plans, using the tables already shown as a template, to begin planning your priority objectives. Create two tables: one headed 'What does your future look like? Months 1–6' and the other headed 'What does your future look like? Years 1–5'.

Insight

Practise exercising the power of your unconscious mind today. Think about an element of your weight loss that you struggle with – perhaps finding healthy snacks is one example – and charge your unconscious mind with finding solutions to this issue. Then go about your day and see what you come up with.

NLP tools to help you stay slim for good

Planning your future

Don't leave anything to chance or circumstance. Take charge of your life.

10 THINGS TO REMEMBER

1 Planning your objectives increases your chances of success.

2 There are potential costs and consequences attached to working on a number of objectives at the same time.

3 Assess your life as a collection of priorities and seek balance with all your objectives.

4 Make conscious plans for your future.

5 Hand over some of your outcome planning to your unconscious mind.

6 Consider your short-, medium- and long-term future.

7 Use your planner to schedule your objectives in a realistic and manageable way.

8 Review your planner regularly and update your objectives.

9 Borrow strategies from one area of your life and adapt them for success in other areas.

10 Using the planner helps allocate time in the most effective way. You should never be too busy to plan. Your planner is the difference between being busy and being effective.

5

There is no failure, only feedback

In this chapter you will learn:
- *how to overcome the fear of weight loss failure*
- *how to pinpoint the most effective behaviour changes to suit your weight loss goals and your personal situation*
- *how to plan a food routine that works for you forever.*

Within NLP there are a number of presuppositions. These are simple statements designed to help us more readily understand the world and the people within it, including ourselves. One of the most powerful of these presuppositions that can be applied to weight management and weight loss is, 'there is no such thing as failure, only feedback'.

The reason this presupposition is so powerful within the context of our attitude to body image, is that when people choose to embark upon a healthy eating routine with specific weight loss objective in mind, they hope to achieve the perfect solution, and they hope to achieve it immediately. If success doesn't come fast enough, they consider this a failure and this notion of 'failure', repeated regularly, as it often is with yo-yo dieting, can be very damaging to our state of mind.

We've already mentioned how important it is to state objectives in a positive manner. This is because if you spend too much time formulating negative thoughts and statements, this is what your mind will focus on and this can lead to behaviour that encourages negative results. To compound this, if you repeat and reinforce negative behaviours on a daily basis, you will merely guarantee further negative results in the future.

The fear of failure

The idea that there is no such thing as failure can free you from all negative thinking. Never again do you need to chastise yourself for having done the 'wrong thing' in the past. Instead, consider all your past actions and current behaviour simply in the context of the results you are experiencing, and how these measure up to the results you'd like to experience. You can then make a plan to modify or refine your behaviour in the future to guarantee success.

Viewing all results as feedback removes the emotion from many situations. It helps reduce the evocative notions of who did what and why and who's to blame, and helps you focus dispassionately on what needs to happen in the future.

The idea of never experiencing failure in the future is very liberating. There are four key emotions that tie together much of what we do and these are anger, sadness, fear and guilt. Each of these four emotions can go hand in hand with the concept of failure relating to weight management. You may feel angry or sad that you feel you've failed to lose weight in the past. It's also very common for people to verbalize feelings of guilt around what they eat and drink, or don't eat and drink, in relation to their weight loss objectives.

It's also extremely likely that one can experience a fear of failure in the future when setting weight management targets. If this were not the case, why hesitate from embracing objectives right away. For many individuals, it's simply the anticipated anxiety they'd experience if they were unable to turn their dreams into reality that prevents them from taking the first steps.

LIFE WITHOUT THE FEAR OF FAILURE

The result of the four key emotions when linked with failure is that negative thinking will lead to negative behaviour or, in many cases, perhaps even total paralysis from taking the action you know you need to take. The fear of failure can be debilitating.

So what if you didn't have to face this fear? Imagine, for example, how different some of the decisions you make on a daily basis might be if you had no fear of failure in the future.

A QUICK CONFIDENCE BOOST

Thinking this way can also do wonders for your confidence. If you are
always concerned about failure, your desire to try new experiences
can become very limited. Knowing there is no such thing as failure
opens up your mind to new possibilities you can experiment with and
then either adopt or reject as part of your ongoing plan for the future.

KEEPING IT SIMPLE: THINKING YOURSELF SLIM

The simple way to think yourself slim for good is to know and
understand what patterns of behaviour lead you to the results
you desire, and then to make sure you follow these patterns
consistently. There is no need to make the process any more
complicated than this.

No failure, only feedback: gathering evidence of what works

As mentioned in Chapter 3, the most reliable way to gather feedback
is to keep a food diary. It also helps to keep an exercise diary or
activity diary as this helps you see the whole picture of energy you
are consuming in relation to energy you are burning off. Using both
these resources you have a detailed record of what your routine looks
like every day, what results you are experiencing and where you can
make changes to modify your results in the future.

Many people make the mistake of waiting for a quiet day or week so
they can focus their attention on spending time making notes of what
they eat and drink, how active they are, and how they can analyse
and interpret this information. One reason why keeping a food diary
during a quiet period can have limited results in the long-term is that
you have far more time on your hands to think about food, buy food,
prepare meals and snacks and get active. So your food diary may end
up being unrepresentative of how food and exercise fit into your life
for the majority of your time.

Healthy eating is often easier when life is quieter, but it has to be maintained when things get busy. Getting active isn't so much of a challenge when you have time on your hands, but it can be trickier when you're struggling to find gaps in your schedule. For the best results with weight management in the long-term, don't wait for a quiet period to begin your diaries – start right away. Note down what you eat and drink in as much detail as possible, along with all instances of exercise and activity. Build up a detailed picture of what's happening right now.

When compiling your food diary you need to note:

▶ what you eat and drink
▶ when you eat and drink these items
▶ how much of any item you eat or drink
▶ how you feel before, during and after you consume any food or drink.

This section can also include a 'hunger rating'. This is a score from one to ten relating to how hungry you are/were when you consumed each item. This will help you build up a picture of the best timing for your meals and snacks. If you find that you are regularly eating when you rate yourself a one, two or three on the hunger scale, i.e. not very hungry, you may wish to space your meals out a little. If you notice that you often feel very hungry when you eat, i.e. an eight, nine or ten out of ten on the hunger scale, you may wish to increase the regularity of your meals and snacks. The danger of feeling too hungry when you eat is that you run the risk of either overeating or selecting options that are high in fat or high in sugar.

It's also a good idea to include an enjoyment or satisfaction rating for each of your meals and snacks to help you monitor what will remain in your routine and what will need to be substituted. If you find that you're eating or drinking items that are neither enjoyable nor satisfying too often, you'll need to make some efforts to replace these items.

You need to keep your food diary up to date under a variety of different circumstances:

▶ at home by yourself
▶ at home with the family
▶ in the office
▶ in meetings
▶ when travelling for work
▶ while commuting

► on holiday
► when socializing.

There is obviously the practical issue of how you ensure that your records are complete, particularly if you spend a lot of time with other people and don't want to appear obsessive about your food. You can make notes on paper, on your phone, on your computer or on your PDA, and then set aside a little time for collating all the information. These days there are a number of websites or phone applications that will help you track your food intake and even calculate calories and nutritional values. If it's easier, simply design a template you can print off and complete periodically throughout the day. There is an example of a food diary template included below.

Sample food diary template

Date	Time	Food/drink consumed	Quantity	Hunger rating	Enjoyment/ satisfaction rating

Experiment until you find the right combination of information gathering techniques to guarantee you have the full picture.

When you have collected detailed records you are in a position to assess your food diary by asking yourself the following questions for each entry:

► Did what I consumed here help me or hinder me in my quest for my ideal body shape?
► Did what I consumed here give me energy or leave me feeling less energetic?
► Did I consume an appropriate portion size here?
► Was this meal or snack high in fat, sugar, salt, or all three?
► Why did I choose these particular options?
► How long did I leave between meals and snacks?

- ▶ Which of these items do I think belong in a healthy eating routine that will deliver the results I am looking for?
- ▶ If I were to remove some items in my current routine, what would I eat or drink instead?

And finally, the ultimate learning question: 'If circumstances were to repeat themselves, what would I do differently that would lead me to a more positive result?'

The other great thing about a food diary is that you can use it to explain many elements of how you feel during the week. If you experience spots of low energy, agitation, loss of focus or difficulty sleeping, chances are these moments will be related to your diet. By looking at your diary you can quickly see the pattern of food items and the timing of meals and snacks that can lead to these symptoms and then plan for alternative strategies that will eliminate the symptoms.

It's also useful to look at the overview of your diary in relation to some common dietary considerations:

- ▶ Am I drinking at least two litres of water a day?
- ▶ Is my alcohol consumption within recommended guidelines?
- ▶ Am I eating at least five portions of fruit and vegetables a day?

By analysing your food diary in this way, you are able to begin developing a picture of exactly what behaviour is leading to current results. Using this information, you can begin planning what would work better than the routine you have currently and what good, consistent, healthy eating looks like for you.

At this point, some of you will be thinking that you're not nutritionists or dieticians, so how will you know what constitutes the right food routine for you?

Be your own healthy eating coach

You'll remember as part of the process of developing well-formed outcomes we looked at ensuring you have the resources at your disposal that you need to achieve your objective. Indeed, another of the presuppositions of NLP is that, 'we have the resources within us to achieve what we want', which means that either we have the knowledge already to ensure success or we can devise ways of acquiring the required knowledge. So if you feel that you need expert guidance, feel free to approach these practitioners. Seeking help is simply a way of being resourceful.

It's also useful to tap into your own resources as much as possible. Healthy eating is not complicated and most of us know instinctively what works well for us and what doesn't. We know what we should eat more of and what we should eat less of. All we need to do is follow our instincts on eating the right things, in the right quantity, at the right time, and do this consistently.

Other useful resources you can utilize are magazines and websites, although there are so many of these resources available that the information can become overwhelming. Target your information gathering to specific topics based on your observations and findings from your food diary. The variety of resources you tap into will become the foundations of your personal plan for success.

Insight

It's great to have access to external advice when appropriate, but to be guaranteed you can always achieve your goals with weight loss, cultivate the notion that you are self-sufficient in your quest to stay slim and any external advice is merely a part of your own efforts. Educate yourself with all the resources you require so you can tap into these resources when necessary, but are never totally dependent on them.

CREATE YOUR OWN HEALTHY EATING GUIDELINES

To help you maintain your healthy eating and weight management routine in the long term, begin compiling some simple healthy eating guidelines that work for you and that you can always keep in mind when making your daily choices. Some examples of generic guidelines are listed below. You can add to this based on your own experiences and experimentation with food.

▶ As a rule of thumb, a meal size should be no more food than you can fit into two cupped hands.
▶ Eat something every three hours. Never leave it more than four hours without eating.
▶ At mealtimes, aim to fill you plate with 25 per cent carbohydrates, 25 per cent protein and 50 per cent fresh vegetables or salad.
▶ Eat slowly, taste and enjoy your food.
▶ Seek out natural food choices that haven't been interfered with too much. Products in bags, boxes, packaging and wraps should be consumed in moderation.

The only way to really know what's in your food is to make it yourself. Make sure that the majority of what you consume is prepared by you rather than in a factory, restaurant or home delivery service.

TRUST YOUR INSTINCTS

Most people have an idea of what they should and shouldn't eat as general principles and also an inkling of what works or doesn't work particularly well for their individual situation. There is a lot of conflicting advice when it comes to low carbohydrate, high protein diet plans, food combining, food for different blood types and food and drink for specific medical conditions. The beauty of the food diary, supplemented with some targeted research, is that it will provide you with the ideal food routine for your specific aims, body type and life circumstance. There will be no more trying to follow different diet books now that you are developing your own, fully customized approach.

THE WEIGHT LOSS QUICK FIX

Keeping a food diary is the most effective way to make the transition from the food routine that you have in place at the moment, that doesn't bring you the results you're looking for with your health, fitness, weight management and confidence, towards the food routine that brings you success in every area of your life. It can also help you attain the holy grail of weight loss – quick and lasting results.

What are you aiming for?

To help in your quest to bridge the gap between where you are now and where you want to be with your food routine, it's a good idea to keep in mind your idea of what 'good' looks like when it comes to healthy eating. This is the time to focus your thoughts on the food routine you imagine yourself following in the future. The more you can practise calling this routine to mind, the easier it will be to reach it in reality. Having a notion of what you think ideal eating looks like will also help you manage your expectations of how close you can get to 'perfect' eating for you within your everyday routine, and taking into account all other considerations and commitments in your life. Here's a suggestion of what good could look like. This is a draft schedule based on one person's routine and objective, and you can modify it to suit your requirements and tastes.

A suggested food routine

	Sunday	Monday	Tuesday	Wednesday	Thursday	Friday	Saturday
Breakfast	Grilled bacon with eggs & wholemeal toast	Porridge	Cereal	Muesli with fruit & seeds	Porridge	Cereal	Muesli with fruit & seeds
AM snack	Free choice	Oatcakes & nut butter	Crackers & low-fat soft cheese spread	Oatcakes & nut butter	Crackers & low-fat soft cheese spread	Oatcakes & nut butter	Crackers & low-fat soft cheese spread
Lunch	Café/Deli sandwich & 1 × fruit	Sandwich & 3 × fruit	Sandwich & 3 × fruit	Sandwich & 3 × fruit	Sandwich & 3 × fruit	Sandwich & 3 × fruit	Café/Deli sandwich & 1 × fruit
PM snack	Free choice	Crispbread & hummus	Nuts & dried fruit	Hummus or tzatziki with chopped peppers, carrot, cucumber, celery	Nuts & dried fruit	Ryvita & cheese	Hummus or tzatziki with chopped peppers, carrot, cucumber, celery

	Sunday	Monday	Tuesday	Wednesday	Thursday	Friday	Saturday
Evening meal	Roast chicken with vegetables and potatoes	Spaghetti bolognese or chilli con carne	Fish with jacket potato and vegetables	Pasta bake	Fish, potatoes, salad	Pork chops and vegetables	Chicken curry with rice and vegetables
Supper	Crispbread & nut butter	Crispbread, cheese, grapes	Crispbread & nut butter	Crispbread, cheese, grapes	Crispbread & nut butter	Crispbread, cheese, grapes	

This is not a food routine that would suit everyone, but you'll see that the idea of starting with a template to work towards makes life easier. You no longer have to think about every meal or snack just as you are about to prepare it. The difficulty for many people with a busy routine is that they begin to think about their next snack or meal just a few minutes before they are supposed to be eating it, which will instantly limit the choices that they have. Or, worse still, they begin to think about food just after the time when they should have eaten it which means that they are over hungry and will naturally be drawn to options that are high in sugar or fat, or will simply eat too much of whatever they can get their hands on.

Following a schedule similar to this one means that you know what meal choices are coming up and you can plan to have the necessary items in stock at home or available where and when you need them. This makes shopping trips quicker, your daily routine more straightforward and evening meals much more organized, as you'll never be caught out wondering what to eat, drink or cook.

A BALANCED FOOD ROUTINE

Think about the balance of your ideal food routine, particularly where some meals and snacks feature regularly and others just once a week. For most people, some repetition in a plan is good as it means you don't need to consider different options every single day. A degree of variety is also important to prevent you becoming bored with the routine. This balance varies for all individuals. Some people love to follow a fixed plan every single week. The familiarity and routine makes life easy for them. Others are put off by what they perceive to be the monotony of a lack of variety, so their food routine needs to change regularly. No approach is either right or wrong, but it will be important for you to decide which approach is best for you so you can plan your schedule accordingly.

Insight

To work out which style of scheduling will work best for you, think about your behaviour in other areas of life. If you take the same holidays to the same places year after year, you're probably someone who benefits from familiarity. If you always seek out new destinations and adventures, you may be bored with a food routine that has too much repetition.

Planning exactly what good looks like also tells your brain that you will, sooner or later, arrive at a situation where you are sticking to what good looks like and living with the food routine that suits your every need. This also helps to speed up the process of establishing the routine that works for you. If you can describe your ideal food routine that will work at some time in the future, why not put it into action, right now? Start with the ideal and use your food diary to observe how this routine suits you and what modifications you need to make to arrive at a practical everyday pattern. Use the sample suggested food routine shown earlier to create your first version of what successful healthy eating looks like for you.

DEVELOP FLEXIBLE OPTIONS

When you have your initial thoughts on what good looks like, you'll be able to highlight specific days when you can put your plans into action. Remember though, the speed of your success with healthy eating will depend on your ability to be flexible.

Despite the best intentions, some people can be knocked off track by a day of meetings, a day out of the office or a day where the children are ill and they're thrown out of their routine. If this happens it can be a struggle to get back on plan. Sometimes, a single day of interruptions to the ideal food routine can take a few days to recover from.

This isn't the case if you have pre-planned routines and taken account of all possible scenarios you may come across in your weekly schedule. Write down all the resources you need in order to eat healthily through each type of day that you encounter in your routine and then check your forthcoming diary to ensure that you have access to everything you need for the week to come, regardless of what that week looks like and where you'll be. Then simply follow your pre-planned routines. You'll quickly find that thinking about your daily food routine in advance saves you much time and effort later on.

The results of effective planning

Using a food diary and applying the guidelines above, you can very easily achieve results just like those sent to me in an email from one client, Amelia, just 19 weeks after getting started with thinking herself slim for good.

I have lost now more than 11 kg (24 lb), nearly 12 kg (26 lb) in fact. I continue my daily and weekly routine, continue to drink more water and I have noticed that my headaches, which were a real nightmare, have, in very large majority, disappeared.

Of course I continue to go to the swimming pool with my children each week. I try also to maintain a variety of different sport activities (walking, bicycling) and I will progressively start tennis. Those moments are very important not only for me but for my whole family and I couldn't go back on this progress.

Yoga is now part of my weekly routine (twice a week) and my assistant is in charge of planning it in my agenda as she does with my other daily meetings.

The most efficient thing for me is that now I can both have 'working dinners' in restaurants and manage my weight and energy. I know myself and I can feel now when I have to stop eating at each meal and when I have to restore my energy. I drink only one coffee a day and sometimes no coffee at all – compared to the four or five I previously had.

You'll notice a number of interesting things in this report and you can see right away many elements of the well-formed outcome planning and specifying the details of the future that we've covered so far. When it came to deciding what good looked like for the future, Amelia used the feedback from her food diary to plan food options for home, office and when entertaining for work, as well as what quantity of drinks including water, alcohol and coffee would be appropriate for her in the long run. She looked at exercise options that would involve her children, both to make exercise more appealing and therefore more likely to happen, and also to tick the box of achieving more family time while getting slim, rather than thinking that focusing on losing weight had to become such a priority that it created less family time, as had been the case in the past.

You can also see elements of away from and towards motivation in Amelia's journey. Obviously she wanted to move away from the weight she was at the beginning of the process and when asked about circumstances she would like to move towards, she highlighted her ideal weight along with other beneficial changes to her routine, including more relaxation time, more confidence and more control. Finally she mentioned that experiencing fewer headaches would create a real improvement in her quality of life and she began immediately visualizing a life without headaches.

There was also a lot of detail in Amelia's plan, including a focus on how to achieve her goals within a very busy working routine, and attention to the importance of a reliable support network. By following the well-formed outcome strategy, Amelia turned an unproductive food diary into a successful healthy eating routine. By applying the step-by-step process, she moved from a point where she thought that it would be nice to lose a few kilos but couldn't see how she would do it, to a situation where she was so excited by the prospect of achieving this goal and all its associated benefits that she was able to plot a clear strategy and achieve fantastic results in a very short time. At the point I received this email, Amelia was still in the process of further refining her plan for even greater achievements.

NLP tools to help you stay slim for good

No fear of failure

Now you are free to make decisions based on what you want to happen without restricting yourself with the fear of what could go wrong.

Real life evidence

No more guess work involved in deciding what will work. Your detailed records will show you what to do more of and what to do less of.

An understanding of what good looks like

A clear idea of the food routine that will lead to the weight loss results you're looking for saves you time and effort every day.

10 THINGS TO REMEMBER

1 The more detail you can collect about your current food routines, the easier it will be to make the right changes for the future.

2 When you have a detailed record of the routine that leads to sub-optimal results, you can very quickly identify simple changes that will improve your results quickly.

3 By engaging with your food routine you will reinforce the links between what you eat and how you feel.

4 There is no such thing as bad food, simply inappropriate portion sizes or an incorrect balance of food in the routine.

5 Variety is the spice of life when it comes to food choices. Different foods provide you with different vitamins, minerals and nutrients.

6 Once you have consciously planned your food routine, you can follow your schedule with no more thought or time commitment than you currently devote to planning and eating. You will however experience dramatically improved results with your weight loss.

7 There should be no emotion attached to your food diary. Use it to analyse what's going on with your food and to plan more appropriate behaviour for the future. Do not dwell too long on what you think isn't 'right' with the diary. There is no failure, only feedback.

8 Plan in advance food routines for all the different circumstances of your life.

9 Have snack options with you at all times. You wouldn't leave home without your phone and simply hope to be able to make some calls during the day. Similarly don't leave your ability to eat healthy snacks to chance.

10 When you discover the food routine that works for you, every element of your daily life will become easier.

6

....

The Meta Model

In this chapter you will learn:
- *how to answer previously unanswered weight-management questions*
- *how to challenge and update your thoughts about losing weight*
- *how to change your attitude to weight management forever.*

As we have clearly established, by questioning your current way of doing things, you will arrive at a new mode of operating that gets the results you desire. Asking questions of yourself can change your view of your circumstances and NLP has many techniques designed to help you interpret the world around you in new ways and discover fresh perspectives. One such tool is called the Meta Model.

The Meta Model is a technique that examines thought and language. Knowledge of the Meta Model enables us to challenge limiting thinking, provides new information relating to familiar situations, and helps to fill in gaps where information that is crucial to our progress and development may be missing.

The Meta Model can be a particularly useful tool when applied to weight loss or weight management as it provides a further method by which to analyse situations where we are finding it difficult to make the progress we would like to, or where we need to look beyond our initial reactions and responses which could be creating barriers to our success.

The Meta Model includes a variety of analyses of, or challenges to, thoughts and statements that we experience every day. This includes our own thoughts, both those that remain in our head and those that end up as verbal communications, as well as statements that we hear from other people. As you now know and understand, there are many benefits to considering internal and external communication at a deeper level and the Metal Model provides you with a specific framework within which you can move beyond the surface level of any communication and shed new light on many situations.

When we considered beliefs in Chapter 2, we looked at how we may perpetuate outdated beliefs or accept our own assumptions relating to what we believe, almost without question, simply because we have always done so in an attempt to keep life simple. This process, basically a method of filtering and condensing experiences into manageable chunks, can extend to the way in which we engage with language, very quickly resulting in the development of stock phrases, ideas and answers that inhabit our head without question. Remaining in this mindset will mean perpetuating the current state of affairs in every area of your life. So now is the time to think again about every idea you have, statement you make or conversation you engage in. This is where the Meta Model is invaluable.

The Meta Model helps you to analyse certain elements of any communication by picking up on what's said or what's missing in each communication. It provides us with three key themes to look out for in any communication, so we'll examine these themes in turn to familiarize ourselves with them and then take a look at how the Meta Model can be useful in helping you stay slim forever.

The key three themes of the Meta Model are:

1 deletion
2 distortion
3 generalization.

Deletion

Because we are surrounded by a busy world and are constantly bombarded by information and images, the brain has a method of preventing overcapacity by deleting much of the information that we are exposed to. Our brain simply selects what to acknowledge and what to ignore, some of this deletion occurring in the conscious mind and some at an unconscious level. Studies have shown that your conscious mind has the ability to hold seven (plus or minus two) items of information at any given time. Fortunately we have the power to decide which items we choose to focus upon and we do so by continually preparing and updating our list of priorities for our attention. Then, by selecting certain tasks to focus on we push others out of our conscious mind to prevent us becoming overloaded.

Insight

Your unconscious mind can cope with a lot more information than your conscious mind, and is constantly doing exactly that. As you focus your conscious mind on the priorities of the moment, your unconscious mind is at the same time assessing what your next set of priorities should be and continually alerts your conscious mind to thoughts and ideas for consideration, whether it be for consideration now, later today, tomorrow, next week or next month. Your unconscious mind is like the safety net that ensures anything that requires your attention will be dealt with. While you consciously choose your priorities for the day, your unconscious mind assesses your decisions and will alert you and encourage you to reassess these decisions if there is a chance that you might act in a way that isn't in your best interests.

So, throughout each day we are monitoring our surroundings, tuning into certain elements of what's going on in our minds and in the wider world around us, while filtering out many more aspects of daily life.

The elements that we decide to tune in to or ignore will dramatically affect how the day runs, and once you are familiar with the various elements of the Meta Model, you will quickly fall into the habit of noticing and questioning the deletions that you make in order to help each day pass more smoothly. Once you are aware of these deletions, you can begin to challenge them and, by doing so, open up new options and possibilities for how you approach the various challenges and opportunities you face in your routine and what you might be able to achieve each day.

There are four principle ways in which we make deletions.

SIMPLE DELETION

A simple deletion occurs when an important element is omitted from a statement. The missing element could be an object, a person or an event. The result of a simple deletion is that the statement makes sense at a surface level but doesn't offer much scope for engagement or for development of the situation.

This often happens when people are preoccupied by something in their own mind and then embark on a conversation with you by simply launching into their subject as if you are party to their thoughts. 'Oh yes, yesterday was a difficult day'. The deletion needs to be challenged in order to discover what the missing element of the sentence is so that you are in a position to deal with the situation in full possession of the facts. You need to find out the specifics of what it was about yesterday that was difficult.

It is possible to respond to a statement where a simple deletion has been made, and many people do, but there is a risk that you end up with a conversation that's full of guess work on your part and thus quite difficult to sustain, or you end up making sympathetic noises for the sake of it without any chance of moving the situation forward.

COMPARATIVE DELETION

In a statement where there is an implied comparison, but the person making the statement doesn't tell you the context of their observation or the frame of reference they have in mind, you need to establish further details of their thinking before you can respond fully. For example, if someone says, 'I'm so fat', you need to ask who they are comparing themselves to when they make the decision they are fat.

You can find yourself making statements such as this as part of your own thought process and if you do, you should always stop and ask yourself what you are comparing your current situation to, and if this is indeed a fair comparison. Do you think you are fat compared to other people that you know? Do you think you are fat now compared to how you were in the past? Do you think you are fat compared to medical norms charts? Again, it's hard to move this thought process forwards without filling in some of the gaps.

As soon as you know the details of the comparison you are able to turn thought into action. If you think your current position can be negatively compared to someone else, you then instantly have an example of towards motivation that you can work with. It may be true that you're not as thin, rich or happy as someone else, but rather than use their success in these areas as a way to make yourself feel negative, hold them up as an example of something you can aspire to. Take a good look at how they have achieved what they have, and be motivated by their success. If they can do it, so can you.

LACK OF REFERENTIAL INDEX

In these statements, the noun, object, person or event isn't specified. In order to make sense of the statement and come up with solutions you need to discover what is being referred to by recovering the noun. An example is if someone were to say, 'They make my life difficult.' You need to find out who, specifically, makes their life difficult.

'Don't you think the way he behaved yesterday was appalling?' Who is 'he'? What did he do? Which specific element of his behaviour yesterday was appalling? As soon as you have answers to these questions you can begin analysing what went on yesterday and how we learn from it and move on. Without these answers, we're stuck with a simple negative reflection of what took place the day before.

UNSPECIFIED VERBS

In some statements, a verb isn't clearly defined, making it essential to clarify what the situation is in more detail. When it comes to weight management, many people think or say, 'I eat badly,' and use this as the reason why they can't reach or maintain their target weight. This statement is too general to be able to respond with targeted, useful advice. In order to arrive at a more positive situation, one needs to ask, 'in what ways, specifically, do you eat badly?'

Insight

Focusing on violations of the Meta Model breathes new life into what could sometimes be quite dead end conversations or thought processes. Many people make statements that appear on the face of it to simply underline a situation they are unhappy with, or reinforce a lack of ability to get themselves out of their current situation. Statements like this are affirmations of an unhappy present without any attempt to contemplate what would be required to make the future better. These statements are at best quite passive and at worst, negative. Using the Meta Model, both on others and on yourself, means you always have more questions, and more questions lead in turn to more answers.

Distortion

Given the fact that we are continually attempting to simplify the world around us to help us make sense of it, it's no surprise that we can sometimes end up with a distorted view of what's going on. This can in turn lead us to form opinions and conclusions that may not be accurate, but are based on our desire to contain our experiences at a level that helps us feel in control.

While simplifying the world around us can be a successful strategy, it's a good idea to remain alert to when these distortions may actually make life more difficult. The desire to maintain control and understanding of what we know, or think we know, can sometimes mean that we distort the world in a way that limits our chances of development. Some common NLP examples of distortion are listed below.

CAUSE AND EFFECT

This is where a concrete and causal relationship is implied, even though it may not necessarily exist. For example, when considering certain food products, people often say they don't eat a specific item because 'it makes me fat'. But what lies beneath this statement? How, specifically does this food make you fat? Can any item of food really *make* you fat? Would any quantity of this item make you fat? Can this food really be held responsible as the cause of you thinking yourself to be fat?

MIND READING

Mind reading occurs when someone claims to know what someone else is thinking, for example, 'I know they think I'm overweight.' How can anyone know what someone else thinks? What are you basing your interpretation of events on? What evidence do you really have that they think you're overweight? What effect does you thinking that they think you're overweight have on your state of mind?

Insight

If you find yourself indulging in a bit of mind reading, pause for a moment to consider the specific thoughts you are attributing to other people. Are they positive or negative? It's amazing how common it is to mind read negative ideas, 'This person thinks I'm annoying,' 'I know so and so doesn't like me,' but how often do you experience a positive mind read? How often do you find yourself thinking, 'This person seems to really like me,' *or* 'This person seems genuinely interested by what I have to say'? Why do you think you are more likely to opt for the negative mind read? What does this say about you? Are you able to redress the balance slightly?

COMPLEX EQUIVALENCE

In some sentences, two different experiences are claimed to be part of the same things, for example, 'I ate chocolate today – I'm a complete failure.' You need to ask, how does eating chocolate make you a failure? Is there really a link between these two events?

Can you really be sure? Are there any other factors involved here? By what thought process have you linked this event and the conclusion it has brought you to? Are there any circumstances under which eating chocolate does not leave you feeling like a complete failure?

LOST PERFORMATIVES

A lost performative occurs where an opinion is expressed as a fact, for example, if someone were to say, 'It's not possible to maintain a healthy eating plan when you also have to manage a career and a family.' The challenge to a statement such as this would be, 'not possible according to whom?' Or, 'Is it really *never* possible to maintain a healthy eating plan within a busy schedule?'

Statements like this make our lives easier in so far as they help us to console ourselves as to why we're not experiencing the results we would like. They also mean we don't have to attempt to change. They are not however particularly useful when working out how to move on from this situation and achieve our desired results. By challenging the lost performative, you immediately move something from being a firm and 'real' obstacle, and turn it into a temporary stumbling block that you are able to navigate your way around. Your firm opinion of the past becomes a statement that you are now able to assess in a different way.

NOMINALIZATIONS

In these sentences, a verb has been made into a noun, for example, 'There's too much procrastination,' or 'There's too much information.' Challenge these statements by asking, 'Too much procrastination or information about what?' 'How does the fact that there is 'too much' procrastination or information help you or hinder you with your current objectives?'

Generalization

Just as we delete information, we also make generalizations based on previous experience to enable us to form opinions or take action in the present. As with the other elements of the Meta Model, generalizing can be very helpful but it can also lead to a restricted view of the world if not monitored carefully. Watch out for the following.

UNIVERSAL QUANTIFIERS

This is where a broad generalization is made using words like 'all', 'every', 'everybody', 'never', 'always'. This can lead to a very limited view of the world so you must check yourself for evidence with which to challenge these generalizations. If someone says, 'I find it impossible to eat healthily because I hate all vegetables', you must ask, 'Do you really hate every single type of vegetable? Are there any vegetables that you don't hate? Does hating vegetables mean that you can't eat healthily?'

MODAL OPERATORS OF NECESSITY AND POSSIBILITY

These statements can limit our options by using words such as 'can', 'can't', 'should', 'must', 'ought', and 'necessary'. It's important to identify the thinking behind these statements, for example, someone may state something as a necessity, 'I must eat healthily every single day' and by doing so put themselves under a pressure that they can't live up to. When it comes to healthy eating, aiming for perfection can make the job more difficult so the challenge here is to establish what would happen if this person didn't eat healthily every single day? Would this necessarily mean they didn't lose weight? Is there an option to eat healthily for the majority of the time and relax a little at other times? Similarly, someone may say, 'I won't lose weight because I can't exercise' to which you could respond, 'What stops you?', 'Is there any kind of activity you can do?' or 'What would happen if you could exercise?'

PRESUPPOSITIONS

In these statements, more detail is required to make sense of the statement, so it's necessary to clarify what exactly is being presupposed. For example, 'If they liked me they'd make things easier for me.' To which you can respond, 'How do you know they don't like you?' How do you know that if they did like you they would make things easier for you? 'What evidence do you need to see to believe they do like you?'

method of breaking down perceived barriers and devising creative solutions to challenges of all sizes. Initially, operating this way may seem time-consuming and can feel like hard work, so pause for a moment to consider this reaction. Taking the short-term view of keeping life simple has led us to our current situation, be it good, bad or indifferent. If that current situation isn't right for you, for whatever reason, choosing the option to engage at this deeper level is the only strategy that can guarantee optimum results for the short-, medium- *and* long-term.

The Meta Model and the NLP diet

To think yourself slim for good, there's no real need to get hung up on the specific component parts of the Meta Model and the names of each of the elements, but it is valuable to be aware of them and tune into them in your everyday communications. If you do, you'll find the model really does open up new ways of thinking when it comes to devising the mindset you require for consistent healthy eating and successful weight management.

To illustrate the value of the Meta Model and knowledge of when to employ it, consider the likelihood of success with long term healthy eating and weight management if you regularly 'violate' the Meta Model with your own thoughts and attitudes. Take a look at the following three statements:

> *I'm overweight but it's easier to leave things as they are.*
> *Diets are all very well but I'm not good with change.*

> *My life makes me fat. I know everyone thinks that I need to lose weight but I can't do it, I'm so weak. It's more important to be focused at work than it is to spend time worrying about your weight. There's too much thinking to do.*

> *My weight is a constant distraction. I never stop thinking about it. I have to fix the situation now, once and for all. I can't go on like this. Everyone needs to support me more.*

With thoughts like these inhabiting your head, how hard or easy do you think it is to lose weight? Let's take each statement in turn and apply the Meta Model so we can analyse each sentence and dig down into what further questions would help challenge these thoughts and overcome them.

DELETIONS

I'm overweight but it's easier to leave things as they are.
Diets are all very well but I'm not good with change.

Think about all that's missing from just this short sentence.

Simple deletions
If you weren't overweight, what would you be? What would be
better than being overweight?

Comparative deletions
'Overweight' compared to what and compared to whom? 'Easier to
leave things as they are' than to do what instead? How, precisely,
are things now and is it really easier to leave every aspect the same
than to make any change whatsoever? In what ways would things be
different if you didn't leave things as they are? What level of effort
would really be involved in making some simple changes that would
help you achieve your objectives?

Lack of referential index
Which 'diets are all very well'? Which diets or food plans have you
tried? How specifically did they work or not work? How long did
any good results last? The last question is a crucial one because, in my
experience, no one sets out on a healthy eating routine hoping that
the results will be fantastic over a short-term, or even a medium-term
period and then they're happy for things to begin moving in the wrong
direction. Yet this is what people often settle for when they say things
like, 'I followed a plan in the past – Weight Watchers, Atkins, low GI –
and it worked for a while, but then the weight started to creep up again.'

If a healthy eating routine worked, but only for a given period of time,
then it's not the final solution. Your definitive healthy eating plan
will produce results that are consistent for weeks, months and years
to come. Diets may be 'all very well' but until you've replaced this
thought with something more robust along the lines of 'Healthy eating
is a simple part of my daily routine that I want to maintain, because
I know it works for me,' you'll be limiting your chances of success.

Unspecified verbs
How, specifically, are you not good with change? Do you find all
change difficult? Have you ever experienced change that was easy
to deal with?

My life makes me fat. I know everyone thinks that I need to lose weight but I can't do it, I'm so weak. It's more important to be focused at work than it is to spend time thinking about your weight. There's too much thinking to do.

Cause and effect
How, specifically, does your life make you fat? What aspects of your life are making you fat? Are there any elements of your life that don't contribute to making you fat?

Mind reading
How do you know that everyone thinks you need to lose weight? Do you really believe that everyone gives your weight that much consideration? Could it really be the situation that *everyone* thinks you need to lose weight? If you begin to discount the people that don't actually think you need to lose weight, who are you left with? How would it change your perspective if you didn't know that everyone thinks you need to lose weight?

Complex equivalence
How does not losing weight contribute towards you being weak? Are you always weak? Is there anything you do in life where you don't feel weak? Can you make a list of all the reasons why you think you are weak?

Lost performatives
Who says it's more important to be focused at work than it is to spend time worrying about your weight? Have you considered that it may be possible to achieve success with your weight and remain focused at work? What about the possibility that achieving your weight loss objectives could make you more focused at work?

Nominalizations
What, specifically, do you need to think about? How long do you think you need to think about these things?

GENERALIZATIONS

My weight is a constant distraction; I never stop thinking about it. I have to fix the situation now, once and for all. I can't go on like this. Everyone needs to support me more.

Universal quantifiers

Is your weight a constant distraction? Are there any times of the day when you don't think about your weight? What specific thoughts go through your mind when you think about your weight? Are all your thoughts negative? If you think about your weight a lot, are there more positive thoughts you could generate that would help you achieve your goals?

Modal operators of necessity and possibility

What would happen if you didn't fix the situation now? Will there be no other opportunities to fix the situation in the future? What would happen if you were to continue as you are?

Presuppositions

How do you know that everyone isn't being supportive now? How would you know if they were being more supportive? In what ways would more support help?

Checking ourselves and monitoring our language and thought patterns is vital to achieving the things in life we say we want to achieve. Challenging statements forces us to open our minds to alternative possibilities. The difficulty some people face when it comes to losing weight, for now and for good is that they feel they've lived with the issue of needing to lose weight for so long, they are convinced they know everything there is to know about the subject. Indeed, I heard it just the other day: 'I know everything there is to know about being on a diet.' Well that's fine, but do you know everything there is to know about losing weight and staying slim for good? The result of letting thoughts and communications go unchecked is that we risk reinforcing limiting thought processes that have stifled progress in the past, and which will inevitably lead to a further lack of results in the future.

Evoking the challenges contained within the Meta Model forces a new way of thinking, one that removes many limitations and opens up the possibility that at the very least we have a choice about the way we think. We soon come to realize that things needn't be as they have been in the past and that there are instead a multitude of ways in which things can be different for the future, simply by us adopting a new attitude to what at first feels like a very familiar situation.

The unconscious mind

We mentioned earlier in the chapter that, while your conscious mind may be limited in how much information it can hold and process at any given time, your unconscious mind can be a much more valuable resource for achieving what you want in life. Learning when to use either part of your mind, and how to manage both to best effect, is a great skill. For some tasks you'll need total conscious engagement to reach the right conclusion. For other tasks you will benefit from handing over the project to your unconscious mind and waiting for the solution to present itself. You'll know the solution has arrived when you experience a eureka moment. These moments feel as though you suddenly come up with an answer from out of nowhere but really, they are the moments when your unconscious mind chooses to deliver a solution to your conscious mind.

GUT INSTINCT

One important aspect of your unconscious mind is the way in which it alerts you to factors that could be relevant to your overall success. Those moments where you pick up on something but you're not sure why, or even sometimes not quite sure what it is that you're picking up on, are examples of your unconscious mind pushing something up into your conscious mind for consideration.

On a practical level, when it comes to weight loss, these moments are usually when you have a flash of concern or suspect that something or someone or any given situation may cause an issue with your weight loss at some time in the future. When you experience these moments, tune into them. If you can overcome these anticipated potential pitfalls in advance with careful thought and planning, you'll find them much easier to deal with if they crop up in reality. With your new knowledge of the Meta Model you may find that many instances when you felt a sign from your gut are examples of when the Meta Model could have been employed. Your gut instinct is your unconscious early warning system. Learn to recognize its input so you can challenge your thoughts and use the answers you come up with to your advantage.

The Meta Model

A sure-fire way to see opportunities to develop and evolve solutions where before you may have seen only obstacles to your progress.

Your unconscious mind

Take the pressure off your conscious thinking by handing over key tasks to your unconscious mind. The more you do this, the more effective the process will become.

Your gut instinct

Practise tuning into the signals from your gut instinct and you will find that you will always be able to act in the way that you know will lead you to the best outcome.

10 THINGS TO REMEMBER

1 We are continually bombarded by thousands of pieces of information. We filter out much of this to prevent feeling overwhelmed.

2 Our unconscious mind is continually processing a vast range of information while our conscious mind focuses on a few tasks at a time.

3 The language patterns we use help make sense of the world. Sometimes we need to challenge familiar patterns to bring new insights to our daily situations.

4 In every thought or communication you experience, consider the information that could be missing from the communication as much as the information that is present. This will help you formulate questions that will provide you with new insights.

5 Your gut instinct is like your own personal in-built early warning system. Practise making good use of it.

6 Take nothing at face value. Get into the habit of looking beneath the surface level of all thoughts and communications to establish the underlying emotions, motivations and purpose.

7 Updating your thoughts and verbal communications is the first step towards new behaviours that will help you achieve your weight management objectives.

8 Listening more carefully and analysing the verbal communication of others is the first step towards uncovering the true meanings behind what they are saying and is a great way to learn how to challenge your own way of thinking.

9 Keep a written record of how you gradually transform your outdated thoughts and speech patterns and replace them with new ways of communicating with yourself. This long list of positive thoughts that you know are designed to ensure your

reach your weight management objectives will become the foundation of the attitude that will lead you to success.

10 Encourage others to analyse their thoughts and communications. This leads to more carefully considered dialogue and swift resolution of any issues that may affect your success with staying slim.

7

Staying slim for good: see it, hear it, feel it

In this chapter you will learn:
- *how to use the power of your senses to ensure lasting weight management*
- *how you prefer to learn new information and how this knowledge can be used to your advantage with weight loss*
- *techniques to add clarity to your desired future and strategies to make this future a reality.*

The Meta Model is yet another example of an NLP approach that can be applied in many different circumstances. It's one application of the fundamental NLP notion of questioning everything and delving beneath the surface of initial thoughts and reactions, and the well rehearsed responses that we all fall back on during the course of each day.

The reason why this questioning is important is that without it we run the risk of becoming a victim of current circumstances. We can fall into the trap of thinking that our current thoughts and views are an accurate interpretation of the way the world is.

In actual fact, although the physical make up of the world we live in is fundamentally the same for every individual on the planet, the personal world in which each of us operates is very, very different. It would be easy to assume that we all interpret what we see around us in the same way, but this could turn out to be a dangerous assumption, which can severely limit your progress through life.

Cultural differences are one prominent example of the extremely diverse ways some actions or events can be interpreted. While sitting with your feet on the table can represent relaxation in one culture, in another this can be interpreted as the height of rudeness. But what about less obvious examples of how the world is interpreted differently by different people? And how can further understanding of this notion help with weight loss and weight management?

If you've ever watched news broadcasts featuring eye witness reports, or read different individuals' interpretations of live events, accidents or disasters in newspapers and magazines, you'll be familiar with how people can experience the same events in dramatically different ways. Even within the closest of relationships such as friends, family, siblings and married couples, there can be many differences in the ways in which individuals experience both large scale events and everyday occurrences, and how they interpret and process what's going on around them.

This is due to the fact that there are also different ways in which we all prefer to receive information. A greater understanding of how each of us interprets the world around us, and is able to use our experiences to learn and develop, can pay huge dividends for our future progress, including our results with weight management.

NLP study has analysed how we use our senses to interpret events, and has created a concept known as representational systems. These representational systems describe a further way in which we assess our surroundings and filter information in order to make use of it. There are five representational systems, corresponding to the five senses: visual (seeing), auditory (hearing), kinaesthetic (feeling), olfactory (smelling), gustatory (tasting).

Further study of these representational systems suggests that we all have what's known as a preferred representational system, with the most popular methods of interpreting information being with pictures (visual), sounds (auditory) or with feelings (kinaesthetic).

What's your preference?

You can identify your preferred representational system by thinking about events in your past, your favourite holiday, for example. When you consider this trip, what element of it do you focus on the most? Do you create a picture in your mind of where you were? Do you hear sounds familiar to that location? Do you remember how you felt when you were there? Can you smell the smells of the destination, or do you remember the tastes you experienced while you were there?

Representational systems and the NLP diet

Once you are aware of representational systems, you can begin using this knowledge to your advantage. Let's consider the three most common, preferred representational systems – visual, auditory and kinaesthetic – in a little more detail.

VISUAL

If you are someone who prefers to work in pictures, one of your best sources of knowledge when researching information that will help you put together your most effective plan for your future healthy eating routine will be to read as much as you can.

When planning your outcomes and objectives you'll find it helpful to write down what you want to achieve and keep an ongoing written record of how you are doing. You need to regularly take the time to use the information you have researched to visualize in as much detail as possible, every stage of your progress until you have clear pictures in your mind of what you are trying to achieve. The clearer the picture, the more detail you plan, and the more time you spend imagining your outcomes, the quicker and longer lasting your results will be.

For ongoing motivation, research plenty of images of people you would like to look like and keep these in your eye line as you go about your daily routine. You need as many visual prompts as possible to keep you on track with your objectives. Posting your objectives on the wall or the fridge alongside a list of all the benefits you will experience by achieving your objectives will really help to keep you focused. You can also use pictures to represent these benefits – images of different areas of your life that will be enhanced when you reach and maintain your target weight can be very motivating. You could have images of holidays you'll take, clothes you'll wear and social situations that you'll enjoy being a part of.

To capitalize on 'away from' motivation, keep one or two pictures from when you perceived yourself to be overweight, strategically placed where they will spur you on to positive action. Make sure also that you have a greater number of positive images of yourself in great shape displayed wherever you spend most time. This will regularly fuel your 'towards' motivation.

AUDITORY

If you have an auditory preference, you learn best by talking and by listening. You'd rather hear someone explain information or instructions to you than try to process the same information by reading it. When it comes to studying or enjoying books for pleasure, you prefer audio books to reading. You like to solve problems by talking them through with as many different people as possible, the solutions arising as much from the process of thinking how to transfer your thoughts into words, as they do from the input of those you are conversing with.

When planning outcomes and objectives, those with an auditory preference benefit from announcing their intentions to others. For you a dictaphone is a better way of monitoring progress than a pen and paper. When creating the future, think about the sounds you will hear when you have achieved your objectives and consider in great detail the conversations you will have, what you will say to other people and what they will say to you, and about you, regarding your achievements.

Audio prompts, be they inspirational readings committed to CD or podcast, as well as positive internal mantras, are a great way to remain motivated from day to day.

KINAESTHETIC

You may have a kinaesthetic preference and, for you, what matters most is how you feel. This includes physical feelings, sensations and touch, as well as emotional feelings. Those with a kinaesthetic preference aren't too worried about how an object or a situation looks or sounds; what you would really like to do is touch it, experience it or try it on for size to interpret how you feel about it.

When focusing on future weight loss success, think about how you will feel in your new clothes and the confidence your achievements will give you. For kinaesthetic people, planning the future is like trying on a new outfit.

It can take a little bit of time to future plan all sensations and emotions, so processing feelings can be slower than processing pictures or sounds, but only by exploring the full range of positive feelings that will result from making progress will you be able to plan the right approach for you and then follow it through. If this is your preferred representational system, make sure you always allow yourself sufficient time to settle into and fully experience current events or plans for future success.

AN ADDITIONAL APPROACH

There is an additional method by which we interpret information, not strictly a representational system but a process which makes use of the visual, auditory and kinaesthetic representational systems in various degrees to filter the world and arrive at interpretations and decisions that are based on practicality and whether something makes sense or not.

The process is known as 'auditory digital'. If you have a preference for auditory digital thinking you may find it useful to make lists of the pros and cons of a number of options and outcomes. You may visualize scenes from the future, imagine future sounds or establish how you will feel in specific future situations and then make a decision on how to proceed based on which option makes more sense to you and which seems to be the most sensible or practical way to proceed.

If you have an auditory digital preference you will benefit from setting very clearly defined targets for weight loss, reduction in body fat and aspirational clothes that you want to fit into, and then revisiting these regularly judging your progress very specifically by simply assessing whether or not you reach your target numbers or clothes, and then adjusting your plan accordingly to ensure you achieve the next set of targets. If your targets take a little longer to achieve than anticipated, you won't get upset about why but you will want to understand what has happened so you can do things differently in the future.

Understanding representational systems is key to understanding your own behaviour and to discovering the most consistent strategies for your success with your weight loss. Knowledge of representational systems helps you to interpret data and 'translate' information into the language that suits you. Without this translation process, your chances of success can be severely compromised.

Having knowledge of the concept also helps you to tap into all of the representational systems to help you better deal with some situations and encourage a greater likelihood of success. For example, if you are good at visualizing but still haven't achieved your weight loss objectives, try verbalizing what you would like to achieve more often and discussing possible routes to success with other. If you have a kinaesthetic preference, try tapping into the auditory digital way of thinking. This will allow you to remove some of the emotion attached to your weight loss journey and see it more from the angle of a project that needs to be completed. This way you'll be able to focus on the actions required, rather than trying to deal with all the emotions associated with these actions or the inability to perform them consistently in the past.

> **Insight**
>
> Practise tapping into the full range of representational systems as often as you can. Doing so will both help you explore all aspects of any current situations you find yourself in and also enable you to plan all possible outcomes of your future. The more detailed your planning is at this stage, the smoother your path to making your desired future a reality will be.

So what does all this have to do with staying slim for good?

As ever, the more you understand about the way you organize your thoughts, the more efficiently you can go about experiencing healthy eating success. An awareness of representational systems is a means to fast tracking your weight loss results in a number of ways.

1 Research
   Knowledge of representational systems ensures you gather information on how to eat healthily and manage your weight in the way that will help you take quickest action. You can decide to research by reading, listening or doing, based on your understanding of how you receive information most effectively.

2 Motivation
   When motivating yourself every day to positive action that will support you in your weight management aims, you can tap immediately into the sense that will spur you into action. Daily visualization will enhance the detail of what you want to achieve

and help make it a reality sooner. A daily dialogue around your objectives will help you clarify your thoughts and offer new insights into what you can do to speed up your progress. Testing out future feelings on a regular basis will help reinforce your desire to experience these feelings for real and will highlight new strategies to increase the chances of this taking place sooner rather than later.

3 Communication
When you understand representational systems you will find it easier to communicate with others and this clear communication will pay dividends when it comes to losing weight. For successful weight loss you need a clear objective and you also need to ensure that you have a support network in place and that everyone is with you on your journey. The ability to communicate clearly with these people helps to create the environment you require for regular healthy eating. This helps to reduce any stress and anxiety that you may be experiencing in relation to those around you, which can be an impediment to your progress.

When two people share the same preferred representational system, conversations and interactions run very smoothly. You can both see very clearly where you are aiming to get to, you hear the same details of the interaction and you both feel the same way about the purpose of your shared dialogue. But what about when you don't see eye to eye? When what the other person is saying doesn't ring any bells with you, or when you're not in touch with their statements?

When two people have a different preferred representational system, it can seem as though they are talking at cross purposes; sometimes even as though they are speaking different languages. Those with a visual preference think and speak very quickly. Because they work in pictures, which are instant, they can process information very fast. Those with a kinaesthetic preference often require more time to consider a situation as they need to calculate how they feel about things and this takes longer than simply creating a picture in their mind. Those with an auditory preference often find clarity on a situation merely by thinking about it out loud. If their audience is someone with an auditory digital preference, this interaction can be frustrating. The auditory digital person is looking for opportunities to weigh up the pros and cons of the other person's dilemma while the auditory person is simply looking for a sounding board; a pair of open and willing ears they can talk at while they organize their thoughts.

You can identify a person's preferred representational system by the language they use. Once you have identified the preference of the person you are trying to communicate with, you can alter your language slightly in order to speak to them in the way they can most effectively process the information. Listen out for keywords, which are known as predicates, as a way to work out the preferred representational systems of those who you spend time with. A selection of these predicates or clues is provided below.

Language used by those with a visual preference
Let's see how this looks, we'll see, I'll change my focus, how does this look to you, you can clearly see how this will work, I have this result in my sights, what's your view of this situation? Can you shed some light on this? I'm struggling to get some perspective on this matter, I can clearly picture that, can you show me? I'll watch you in action, could you enlighten me?

Language used by those with an auditory preference
Sounds good to me, that rings a bell, listen up, I didn't tune in to what they were saying, we clearly weren't on the same wavelength, I told you, they just didn't hear what I was saying, she mentioned that, I'll ask him, let's discuss this in more detail, talk to me, he's very vocal, she's very quiet.

Language used by those with a kinaesthetic preference
Hot, cold, loose, tight, uncomfortable, comfortable, squirm, move, solid, flaky, pressure, weight of expectation, it feels as though a burden has been lifted, that film touched me, her story moved me, rough, smooth, light, heavy.

Language used by those with an auditory digital preference
That makes sense to me, it's logical, I believe, I perceive, I think, I wonder, I'm not sure how to decide, I appreciate the situation, can you comprehend this? Pros and cons, advantage and disadvantage, positive and negative, taking everything into consideration.

Let's think about this information specifically in relation to healthy eating and staying slim. Consider this dialogue.

Husband: What do you fancy for dinner tonight?

Wife: I feel like I need to lose a few kilos so I'm going to have fish and salad. You can have whatever you fancy.

Husband: Another diet! I can't see why that's necessary, you don't need to lose weight.

Wife: Well, maybe I don't need to but I'd feel a bit better about myself if I did.

Husband: Well, how long is this regime going to last? You know these phases don't seem to make much difference to how you look in the long run.

Wife: I'm not sure. I know what you mean though; it's been on my mind for a while that I need to crack this once and for all. The longer I leave it the more the pressure grows to finally find a solution that lasts, so I'm determined to get it right this time.

Husband: You know my view. If you haven't managed it by now, it's probably not something you should keep looking at.

Wife: It'll be a huge weight off my mind if I can manage it though.

Husband: OK, but I can't see it happening myself.

You'll notice that the conversation isn't smooth and it certainly isn't productive. At times it appears almost confrontational. The husband clearly expresses a preference for visual language and is also quite auditory digital in his preference for decision-making regarding his wife's continued attempts at weight loss. The wife is using kinaesthetic language. How different the conversation could have been if, observing her husband's preference, the wife could have modified her language to better enable him to understand her position.

Husband: What do you fancy for dinner tonight?

Wife: I feel like I need to lose a few kilos so I'm going to have fish and salad. You can have whatever you fancy.

Husband: Another diet! I can't see why that's necessary, you don't need to lose weight.

Wife: I thought I'd have one more focused effort and see how I get on.

Husband: Well, how long is this regime going to last. You know these phases don't seem to make much difference to how you look in the long run.

Wife: Well, I often get so blinded by all the information out there that I lose sight of what I'm doing.

Husband: You know my view. If you haven't managed it by now, it's probably not something you should keep looking at.

Wife: I'm going to begin with a blank canvas this time, change my perspective and take a longer term view of how this needs to work.

Husband: OK, I see. That appears to be a plan that could work good luck. I'll do what I can to help and let's see how it goes.

Think about conversations you've had in the past with your partner, family or friends where you may have felt them to be unsupportive of your weight management objectives. Consider their preferred representational systems – you may be able to identify them already or you may need to spend some time listening carefully to the language each person uses – and then think about how you could make any similar conversations run differently in the future.

> **Insight**
>
> Remember that when discussing preferred representational systems, they are just that, preferred. We all have the capacity to work with all systems and sometimes, particularly when it comes to communicating with others, it's a good idea to practise working with the representational systems that you don't feel so comfortable with. This enables you to switch seamlessly between preferences and make yourself understood by whoever you are communicating with.

Submodalities: creating the details of your future

Knowledge of preferred representational systems also helps with your planning of the future. You already know that the more detail you can add to your thoughts of the future, the more quickly your planned future will become a reality. The clarity of your planning can be controlled by your use of what are referred to as submodalities; the finer details of your imagination.

If you are a visual person, you can determine the power of your visualizations by adjusting the appearance of the images in your imagination, just as you are able to when you watch television, for example. You can turn up the colours, the brightness and the sharpness of the images that you are creating. Make them bold, vibrant and striking. The clearer you can make your visualization, the easier it will be to make this visualization a reality. Pick the size of the screen on which you play your future on carefully. It may help if you visualize everything you want to happen in the future on a large screen so you can see more detail and even step into your visualization so you can experience the perspective of living your future through your own eyes.

For any perceived barriers or obstacles to your progress, visualize the times these events could take place and shrink the images down to a smaller size. Remove the colour from these obstacles, blur the edges of the images and turn down the brightness. By mentally reducing the impact of these troublesome events, you make them less likely to knock you off track in reality.

Auditory people can turn up the sounds of success associated with healthy eating; make them clearer, stronger and more frequent. You can also reduce the noises associated with interference in your healthy eating progress.

For those who prefer a kinaesthetic representational system, you can enhance your future results by becoming more deeply absorbed in the feelings and emotions of anticipated future outcomes.

A belief in NLP is that the mind cannot tell the difference between a real and an imagined experience, which means that we are all capable of calling to mind all the emotions we would associate with a particular event, even if the event doesn't actually take place.

We are able to empathize with the sad events that happen to other people in the same way that we can imagine feelings of great happiness. We don't have to actually lose a job or a loved one to imagine in great detail how that would feel, nor do we need to get a promotion, find the partner of our dreams or win the lottery to imagine what we would go through, mentally and physically, were these events really to take place.

Use this knowledge to maximize as many clear details of the future you would like to live, while minimizing the impact of anything that you think will get in your way. Thinking in this manner will put you in just the mindset you need to think yourself slim for good.

CREATING THE PERFECT FUTURE

To enable you to create the best possible future you can ever comprehend, it makes sense to use the submodalities of all representational systems. This means you create pictures, sounds, feelings, smells and tastes, and for the best possible results, you practise planning your future regularly and in as much detail as you possibly can.

For your plan to become a reality it has to be positive and undiluted by doubts of any description. If you ever feel any doubts creeping into your mind about your ability to succeed, challenge these thoughts until you have reframed them, taken charge of the submodalities, shrunk down all objections or turned them into opportunities which you can then enlarge and take advantage of.

Case study: a light-hearted look at submodalities

Celia had experienced some success with weight loss in the past but, like many people, had also suffered some sideways or backward steps along the way. When she sat down to create a new plan for the perfect weight loss future, she found it quite easy to visualize the scales reading lighter and see herself going about her daily routine wearing new clothes and exuding a confident aura. She could clearly imagine the feelings of achievement and self affirmation triggered by success with weight loss; indeed she had experienced these in the past and so had no hesitation about calling these feelings to mind as an anticipated and regular feature of her future.

Nor did she have any problem anticipating the smells and tastes of weight loss success. Again, she knew from experience that her enjoyment of the taste of everything she ate and drank was vastly improved when she was comfortable that everything she consumed was in line with how she wanted to manage her weight, and she knew all too well that life just smelled sweeter when she was where she wanted to be with her body shape and self image.

Where Celia had come unstuck in the past was that at some point during her weight loss routine, she heard a voice that stopped her in her tracks. Sometimes it was a voice inside her head that questioned her long-term commitment, saying things like, 'You may have done well so far but you've never been very good at sticking to things so it's only a matter of time before the weight creeps on again.'

Or it was the voice of her husband suggesting, in the politest terms possible, that the routine she was following was bound for failure. 'Don't you think you should just go back to eating normally now? After all, you've been on diets like this in the past and you eventually end up back where you started so why don't you just relax about it and eat what you want?' Or it would be the voice of one of her friends saying, 'You can't stay on a diet forever, none of us have managed it, it's just too difficult.'

Because Celia had been knocked off track in the past by such distractions, the voices now began to interrupt even when she was planning how the future would be. She could always imagine experiencing some success with her weight loss but then her planning was always hijacked. The upshot of this was that Celia either behaved consistently with her initial planning process meaning some success, followed by the critical voices causing her some backsliding, or she hesitated with making changes at times where she could potentially have made great progress.

I worked with Celia for a short time during which we broke this cycle by examining the voices and adjusting the submodalities of Celia's future planning. We tried to turn down the volume on the dissenting voices, but because Celia had heard the objections so many times, they kept fighting their way back into her head, so this solution worked at times, but we needed something that worked all the time, without exception. The answer turned out to be the technique of changing the characters associated with the voices.

So, instead of hearing her husband's voice uttering his usual doubting statements, Celia gave him the voice of Donald Duck. To her friends she attributed a variety of comedy characters from David Brent to Vicki Pollard and when she felt her own voice

(Contd)

doubting herself, she changed the tone from a scolding, chiding voice to that of a petulant child. By altering the tone of all the voices that usually affected her mindset, it became impossible to take the doubting and criticism seriously, and increasingly easy to dismiss all objections to anything other than the perfect outcome that she could imagine.

Association and disassociation

Knowledge of representational systems and submodalities can help you plan your weight loss future in an additional way by using the techniques of association and disassociation.

ASSOCIATION

Associating into memories or future plans means experiencing them from the first-hand perspective where you are in the moment, looking out at people and events around you.

To associate into a memory or future plan will heighten its intensity and amplify the emotion. This is a useful technique to employ when you'd like to recapture positive memories or when you are planning positive outcomes for the future and would like to consolidate your motivation to make your plans a reality.

If you've had positive results with weight loss in the past, associate into these memories, as reliving them will spur you on towards experiencing success again as soon as possible.

DISASSOCIATION

Disassociating yourself from memories or future plans means analysing experiences from the second- or third-hand perspective where you are looking at yourself either from the perspective of another person involved in the event, or you are a third party observer of the entire scenario.

To disassociate yourself from a memory or future plan will lessen its intensity and decrease the emotion. This is a useful technique if you'd like to gain a new perspective on the past and move on from negative memories or experiences, or when you are anticipating possible barriers to your success in the future.

If you've had negative results with weight loss in the past, don't try to block out these experiences but instead revisit them with a view to disassociating yourself so that you can learn from what happened and use this knowledge for the future. Change your perspective so you can view your memory through the eyes of someone else who was there, or from the viewpoint of a neutral observer. You cannot change or undo the past but you can use it to grow your knowledge for what lies ahead.

When contemplating what could occur in the future that would block or slow your progress with your weight loss objectives, disassociate yourself from these experiences and you will find that you can quickly devise solutions for dealing with these anticipated moments. We all have the temptation sometimes to take the emotions of the present and apply them to our thoughts for the future, which can limit our positivity or creativity. Where this is a possibility, you can use the technique of disassociation to ensure you judge the future with a clear head and without any limitation that may be part of your current situation.

Perceptual positions

Associating into and disassociating from events is part of the NLP theme of perceptual positions. This technique examines closely the different perspectives we are able to view events from, and the effects on our results that adopting these different perspectives can have.

FIRST POSITION

We all experience our daily routine from first position – looking at the world through our own eyes with our thoughts and decisions filtered and shaped by our personal experience. One limitation of inhabiting first position is that it can result in a lack of perspective. To consider everything that happens to you from this single perspective can lead to a rather one-dimensional interpretation of events and can result in a lack of options in many situations. Fortunately, to help us widen our perspective and keep our options open, we are able to consider the world from different viewpoints.

SECOND POSITION

In any dialogue or interaction, second position is inhabited by the person we are speaking to. By considering how they are reacting to our side of the dialogue, we are immediately better able to formulate our own thoughts. There's a danger that if you only focus on your own thoughts and emotions, you'll be limiting the ways in which you can move forward with any given situation. By putting yourself 'in the shoes' of the other person, you will immediately gain a new perspective on the dialogue, and can then tap into new information relating to the situation that will help you arrive at more positive conclusions.

As with many well-practised routines, there is a positive intention behind the reluctance to move beyond first position. We cling to our view of the world because it helps us understand what's going on around us. To open our mind to the perspectives of others is to invoke a whole new world of questions and uncertainties, which is why it is a skill to be able to do this on a regular basis. Often in our interaction with others we begin the dialogue with an idea of how we would like things to end up and we spend a great deal of time trying to persuade the other person or people that our solution will be the best. If they agree, great. If they don't, we tend to focus on thoughts like, 'Why can't these people see that what I'm saying makes sense?'

The path to a successful conclusion to these communications lies not in digging your heels in and trying more aggressively to persuade people that you are right, but in lightening your grip on your views and opening your mind to considering the motivation behind the thoughts of others and the solutions to the situation that they would prefer. With a greater understanding of their position you are better able to communicate your views and move the conversation forwards in a way that suits all parties.

From a weight management perspective, the ability to adopt second position can be useful when considering why others are behaving in a particular way towards you. If those around you don't respond to you and your objectives as you would like, you can ask yourself, and hopefully answer, questions such as, 'Why is this person advising me to eat or drink this?' 'Why are they reacting this way when I tell them about my weight loss plans?' 'Why do these people appear to be trying to knock me off track? I've told them what I want to achieve but what they're suggesting won't help me at all.'

Put yourself in their shoes for a moment and you can very quickly gain an insight into why they are behaving as they are. Stepping into second position allows you to see yourself as others see you, and this may help you to modify your communications and your behaviour in ways that will help you reach your objectives.

For example, a common complaint from those who are trying to lose weight is that they just don't get the support they require from their partner, family, friends or colleagues. Too much of this can undermine resolve very quickly. From the most positive start, you can quickly fall into a state where your head is inhabited by thoughts such as, 'Why does my partner keep suggesting we eat out, why don't they offer to cook more, why do they always want to eat takeout food, why do they always offer me chocolate, why do they always top up my drink when I say I've had enough?'

Or, 'Why won't my children listen to me when I say we don't need so many crisps and sweets in the house?', 'Why do my work colleagues always bring in cakes to the office?', 'Why do my friends always insist that we go out for dinner rather than just meeting for a quick drink?'

The danger is that you focus on these questions too much and they eventually derail you from the task at hand. They lead you to a place where you end up thinking, 'Well, if everyone else is making it so hard for me to lose weight, perhaps I'll just give up on it for the moment. It's their fault though.'

To avoid being knocked off track by thoughts like this, the first thing to do is to begin answering some of the questions that inhabit your head. Think for a moment about what lies behind the behaviour of others. If you were in their shoes, what would your motivation be in behaving in the way they are behaving? Bearing in mind that the intention of all behaviour is positive, you can be sure that everyone you know has some good intention underlying their actions, even if, at the most basic level, their intentions will be to make their own lives easier or happier. If this is the case, their first step to fulfil this desire will be to try to keep others around them happy and, in many cases, this is achieved by providing for, nurturing or feeding. In short, taking care of the basic needs of other people.

So, while you're thinking, 'Why does my partner keep topping up my drink when I say I've had enough,' they may be thinking, 'I want to ensure that my partner feels loved and looked after and I know that she likes a glass of wine to relax after work. I also know that she thinks she needs to obey the "rules" on how much to drink every evening, but I'd like to encourage her to relax around these rules so I'll just top her glass up for her. She won't do it herself so it'll be a nice thing for me to do.'

Viewing the situation from this perspective can change your response quite dramatically. Rather than thinking that someone's actions are designed to derail you, you can be reassured that they actually have your best interests at heart. You can then explain that the best way in which they can express love and consideration for you, is to acknowledge what you are trying to achieve and then behave in a manner that is consistent with helping you reach your goals. Most people like to be helpful and are happy to receive some guidance on how their positive intentions can best be channelled into actions that result in everyone getting what they want.

A DIFFERENT VIEW ENTIRELY: THIRD POSITION

Third position is the domain of the 'fly on the wall' and is a really useful place to visit if you would like to gain clarity on any decisions, or add an element of calm to any situation where emotions are running high. The world viewed from first or even second position can be quite an intense place. Moving to third position enables you to experience situations as a dispassionate observer, which can be invaluable in managing emotional intensity.

Consider yourself faced with a slice of tempting cake, a pile of your favourite biscuits or a chilled glass of your favourite white wine. You see in front of you just what you're in the mood for, particularly as you've had a stressful day and you deserve a bit of indulgence. You know that this temptation isn't part of today's healthy eating routine, but it looks appealing from where you are right now. In this situation your internal dialogue is in full flow and, chances are, that the argument for short-term pleasure is about to become triumphant.

Pause for a moment and view this situation from third position. Move your perspective outside your mind and body for the moment and see yourself sitting at the table looking at the cake, the biscuits or the wine. Instantly the noise of your internal dialogue should be halted as you're no longer consumed by the intensity of first position but are now outside the moment, looking on. You can no longer feel the urgency of the inner dialogue as you are now an observer of the situation, able to assess the validity of all points of view in a considered way.

As an observer, what do you think about the cake, the biscuits or the wine now? Does the person you are looking at appear to need to give in to temptation? Would eating the cake, the biscuits or drinking the wine make any positive difference to the person that you see? Would they lose anything by not opting for short-term pleasure? What would they gain by opting against temptation?

As a third party observer, how would you advise the person that you see in this situation? What new information comes to your mind as you observe the decision-making process from third position rather than experience it from first position?

As you practise the technique of changing perceptual positions, you will find that moving to third position brings with it a new perspective and calmer insights into any dilemma that you are facing. If there are others involved, third position helps you to imagine how you are being viewed in any interaction and can help with the process of negotiation by allowing you to see how the best mutual solution to any situation can be reached rather than just looking out for what will suit you best as can be the case if you limit yourself to first position.

An important element of achieving your weight loss goals is to follow the plan for success that you have created as consistently as possible and under a variety of circumstances. Sticking to your healthy eating routine is easy when you have full control of all your circumstances. When you can plan, shop, devise recipes, cook and eat at your own pace and under your own control, it can all feel pretty straightforward. Challenges arise as you navigate your way through your daily commitments and obligations, but good planning will always help you stick to your routine when things are busy. The real challenge can come when you introduce other people into the equation.

Third position: a quick way to stay on track
In these situations you may feel compromised in how you'd like to behave. You may feel that whoever is with you may not agree with the way you're behaving in relation to your food routine, so you change your approach according to how you think they will judge you. If you find yourself in this situation, it's important to remember that you don't actually know how your behaviour is being interpreted; you can simply project your own thoughts, which are based on your beliefs and the filters that you place on the world. When you have time, you can apply the techniques we've previously

covered earlier in the book to update these elements of your behaviour if necessary. In the meantime, a quick way to alter how you view the situation is to adopt third position.

If you're concerned that people will judge you for choosing a salad for lunch rather than fish and chips, step outside this situation and view it from third position. Does someone choosing a healthy option over an alternative really result in a critical judgement from others? And if it does, what are the consequences of this? Does it really matter?

If you feel awkward saying no to another bottle of wine when you're out with friends, picture this scene from a neighbouring table or from behind the bar. Is your choice to stop drinking there such a serious one? Is it really likely to spoil the evening?

If you feel uncomfortable making special requests in restaurants so that you can stick with your routine, think about why this is and what you would think if you witnessed the same request from one of your fellow diners. Do you see someone being awkward or do you see someone who knows what they want and is communicating this to someone who needs to know? The way you feel in these situations will be determined by your previous experiences, your beliefs and your values. Changing your view to third position very quickly highlights aspects of your character that you may want to update if you really want to achieve your target weight this time around.

> **Insight**
> Applying your NLP knowledge will ensure that you never feel stuck for options on how to get what you need in any situation. Altering your perceptual position in any circumstances will help you quickly clarify your thoughts and your communication techniques.

Creating your own weight loss future

As ever, your quick success with weight loss depends on full engagement in order to establish specifically what results you want and how you plan to achieve these results, followed by regular review and update sessions to refine your plan of action. Work through the following steps, using the new knowledge you have, and begin getting into the habit of thinking in these terms about your healthy eating routine.

STEP 1: BLUE SKY PLANNING

Regardless of your previous results with weight management programmes, allow yourself the opportunity for a fresh start today. Spend some time working through the details of your desired outcomes. Tap into the sights, sounds and feelings of your life when you have reached your target weight. Take a bird's eye view of all the people, places and environments involved in your future, allow your mind to wander through a variety of scenarios you'll be part of and then float down to associate into these scenarios. This means seeing them through your own eyes, hearing everything around you, experiencing the feelings that go with these scenarios and verbalizing your thoughts and emotions at every stage.

STEP 2: THE DEVIL IS IN THE DETAIL

Continue playing and replaying future scenarios in your head so that you become familiar with every single detail of how things can possibly play out. You may not be able to predict every aspect of future behaviour, particularly where other personalities are involved, but you'll have a good idea of what will happen, and the greater the number of possible outcomes you can rehearse in your head now, the better equipped you'll be to react and think on your feet in reality.

STEP 3: DAMAGE LIMITATION

As you plan your future events, conversations, meetings and daily life in general, thoughts will spring into mind of times when you suspect you'll find living with your healthy eating and weight management routine a challenge. Now is the time to address these situations and decide how you will proceed if they arise. Having a plan for all eventualities will mean you are able to navigate your way through any situation or challenge that arises. Just as you increase the details and clarity around every angle of the future you want to be living, acknowledge your likely challenges, address them from different points of view and then adjust the submodalities of these situations to minimize or remove any possible impact these challenges could have.

STEP 4: CHECK YOUR COMMITMENT

As you imagine your future, the positive feelings that you anticipate should be present right now. These current feelings are an integral part of your forthcoming success. Acknowledge them and assess them. Are these feelings enough to allow you to rate your commitment level to achieving your success as a ten out of ten? If not, what further work do you need to do with your plan for the future in order to be able to say that you're fully and unquestionably committed to success. Without a ten out of ten commitment level, you may be compromising your potential results even at this stage. Revisit any aspect of your future plan that you feel is preventing you from experiencing full commitment.

Do you need to alter the size of your target or change the time frame within which you're hoping to achieve it? Do you need to examine your objectives from a different perspective? Do you need to work on adjusting the submodalities of your future life? Are there specific barriers that you still feel could block you from succeeding with your goal?

Spend a little time exploring all the reasons why you feel you can't score yourself a ten out of ten for commitment and then either deal with these factors right now, or make an action plan with a deadline for each area you need to address so that you know exactly when you'll be able to score a ten. Once you're confident you have total commitment, there will be no reason why you can't achieve complete success, so be quite strict with yourself about taking prompt action to clear the way for a score of complete commitment.

At this stage, if you feel the need or desire to capture the feelings of motivation that you are currently experiencing, do so in the way that you will find most useful to revisit and spur you on when necessary. Write down your aims and all the advantages you'll experience when living with your positive results. Draw sketches or pictures of your future or collect images that you can aspire to for your own situation. Record your thoughts right now on audio tape or on video or write yourself a letter detailing what you want to achieve and why.

STEP 5: LIVE THE DREAM

This means begin living the dream right now, not at some stage in the future. Everything you do, all day, every day, should be consistent and congruent with the result that you want to achieve.

STEP 6: FUEL THE FIRE

Spend time regularly working on the details of your future plan and updating any elements based on your daily experiences. Everything you do will provide you with feedback on your current routine so that you can refine your approach for optimum results in the future. Remain vigilant and observant and make it your mission to seek out people and situations that will provide you with new insights into how best to achieve your chosen weight loss objectives. Use these insights to add yet further detail to your plan.

NLP tools to help you stay slim for good

Representational systems

Analysing thoughts and language for the most effective communication with yourself and others.

Submodalities

Adjust your sensory perception to change how you feel about the past, present and the future.

Association/disassociation

Changing perspectives to enhance the positives and decrease the negatives.

Perceptual positions

Change your perspective to change your results.

10 THINGS TO REMEMBER

1 Understanding representational systems helps you uncover the true meanings of communications.

2 You can instantly increase your rapport with people by speaking to them in their 'language'.

3 Planning your weight loss future using your preferred representational system, bolstered with use of other representational systems will speed up your results.

4 Regular use of all representational systems enhances both internal and external communication.

5 Adjusting submodalities can have a dramatic effect on your interpretation of events.

6 Associate into experiences to heighten intensity.

7 Disassociate from experiences to lessen intensity.

8 Successful weight loss demands clear planning and effective internal and external communication.

9 Remember that everyone 'reads' events slightly differently. Be sympathetic to this in your planning and your communications.

10 Get into the habit of viewing situations from different perceptual positions. Make a mental or physical note of the new insights gained from adopting these positions.

Remove all barriers to staying slim for good

In this chapter you will learn:
- *how to quieten negative thoughts inside your head*
- *how to remain positive at all times*
- *how to make effective weight-management decisions.*

You know only too well by now that NLP focuses a lot of time and attention on how we can do things differently in the future. This concept is where the notion of 'no failure, only feedback' comes from, and it is why NLP techniques encourage us to ask so many questions. Every question that you ask, and of course answer, will equip you with new information for the future. As you practise looking at life through an NLP lens, you'll become more accustomed to this inquisitive way of thinking, particularly as you gather more evidence to convince you that this way of operating greatly enriches your life.

Insight

Take a moment to acknowledge the ways in which you now think differently about your weight management objectives and related behaviours. Write down as many new thoughts and insights that have struck you since you began reading this book as you can. Every new insight you can think of will increase your chances of staying slim for good.

Armed now with an understanding of the Meta Model and the concept of representational systems, you can see how important it is to analyse not only what you experience when communicating with others, but also to question what takes place within your own mind every moment of every day. This, after all, is how we seek to make sense of our lives. We are all continually having conversations in our head and it is easy to see how the tone of these conversations, our inner dialogue, is set by our beliefs, our previous experiences, and the filters and language that we use to judge and interpret daily events. What matters is that we monitor these conversations to make sure they help us in our lives and our quest to stay slim for good, and check that we're not talking ourselves out of potential success.

For most people, the patterns of their inner dialogue become so familiar that they are never questioned. In fact, beyond being familiar, they become comforting over the years. In a world of change, your internal dialogue becomes a safe haven where you can retreat to what you know, take control of whatever is happening around you and put the world to rights.

Inner dialogue and the NLP diet

Our inner dialogue can be a valuable asset in keeping us calm during challenging moments and secure throughout our life, but it can also limit our development if left unchallenged and not regularly brought up to date. This balance between security and personal development is also the basis of most discussions in our head. Consider the following internal dialogue for example.

> *My job has become a bit boring, maybe I should ask about a promotion.*
> **Be careful though you don't want to rock the boat.**
> *But I don't want to be seen as unambitious. Then I'll be stuck doing this job forever.*
> **But what if you end up with a role you can't manage.**
> *I need to push myself a bit.*
> **What if you don't get on with your new colleagues?**
> *Maybe I should try to find a job in a different company.*
> **But this company has a great pension scheme and the location is easy to get to from home.**
> *Who knows what opportunities are out there, I haven't looked around for ages. I might find something even better than the situation I'm in now.*
> **It's a tough job market though, aren't you better staying where you at least have some security?**
> *Maybe you're right; perhaps I should just leave it for a while. Better the devil you know, after all.*

THE ANGEL AND THE DEVIL

The two voices of our internal dialogue are often likened to an angel and a devil. One part of the dialogue can appear to advocate the positive while the other feels as though it's focusing on the negative. One voice argues for change while the other lists all the reasons why you should leave things as they are. One side of the dialogue seems bold and brave while the other is more conservative. One half of you seem to be ambitious while the other half is happier with stability.

> **Insight**
>
> Can you think of any recent examples of an internal dialogue? What was the conclusion of the dialogue? Did you begin to do anything differently following the dialogue?

NLP believes, as we'll see in a moment, that the intention of all behaviour is positive, so it may be more accurate to suggest that one side of your internal dialogue usually argues in favour of changing something now and upsetting the short-term stability in favour of the possibility of achieving a better situation in the medium- or long-term. The other voice argues for leaving things as they are, which, on the face of it, is the solution that offers the least disruption and greatest short-term security. So, rather than a dialogue being positive versus negative, it's more accurate to suggest the dialogue is between short-term positive results and long-term positive results.

Your internal dialogue becomes most animated when you feel that you need to make changes. At this point, the arguments in your head can become quite involved and quite heated and sometimes quite hard to see a way out of. You begin to feel anxious and stressed, just when you need clear thinking the most.

One of the problems when your inner dialogue becomes heated is that sometimes you feel as though you're merely going around in circles. The arguments on either side may have become a little repetitive, you're not hearing anything that you haven't heard before, and there's no new information being brought forth that tells you exactly how to move on from your current dilemma, whatever it may be. You need some new thinking and the first thing you can do to challenge your inner dialogue is to apply the techniques of the Meta Model.

Examine the last example of an internal dialogue regarding changing jobs from the point of view of the Meta Model. See how many unanswered questions there are, how many generalizations and other violations there are; how many options and opportunities there are left unexplored, simply because most of us perceive that it's easier to leave things as they are. Practise your skills with the Meta Model by seeing how many violations you can spot.

The reason we allow ourselves to get away with such circular internal dialogues is that, for the majority of the time, we are sufficiently content with the way things are in our lives to leave them alone. We use our internal dialogue to justify daily decision-making that prevents us from asking too many questions or rocking the boat too much. Sure we have moments of dissatisfaction when we can feel a burst of desire to move away from something that's bothering us, or we feel moments of inspiration and the urge to move closer towards something that has excited us, but often these moments aren't afforded the respect they deserve. These are the times when our unconscious mind is flagging up issues for consideration, which would begin with an internal dialogue. In many cases, however, we push these alerts away thinking we don't have time for them. At these moments, our dialogue can be condensed down into a variation on the theme of, 'That was a bad/good thought/experience, I hope I get less/more of that in the future.' And there we leave it, hoping things will be different tomorrow but happy to carry on as we are for now.

Thinking this way isn't necessarily a problem, but it can inhibit your ability to fulfil your potential in many areas of life. Without tuning in to the signals that are suggesting change may be a good idea, or questioning familiar patterns of thought and dialogue, how can you grow beyond your current situation?

Inner dialogue and staying slim for good

Let's look specifically at how our inner dialogue can affect our results with weight management.

> *Oh my goodness, these trousers feel a bit tight. I really have to lose some weight.*
> **That sounds like a great idea, how shall I do it?**
> *I need to be strict with my food routine.*
> **How much weight do I want to lose?**
> *At least 7 kg (15 lb).*

In how long?

As soon as possible, how about in one week?

That sounds like a tough challenge.

But I'm so fed up with my body; I've got to do something.

OK, what exactly?

Salads for lunch, chicken or fish for dinner, no snacking and I won't bother with breakfast, that should save a few calories every day.

That should all help.

Oh, and I need to cut out wine as well.

And will that all help me reach my goal of being 7 kg (15 lb) lighter in a week?

It might do.

Have I tried a similar approach in the past?

Yes.

Did it work?

No, not really.

What will be different this time?

I really need to make this work this time.

OK, so let's think practically. Will I be having salad for lunch today and a healthy evening meal with no alcohol?

Yes. Well, maybe not today. I'm out for lunch with some colleagues and then meeting a friend for drinks and maybe some food this evening.

How about tomorrow?

Tomorrow could be better but already the thought of a salad for lunch seems a bit dull. Looking forward to lunchtime is the only thing that makes the morning bearable. Then I'm out at the cinema in the evening so will have to grab some food when I can.

OK, how about this weekend?

We're having a dinner party on Saturday night so I know there will be quite a lot of food involved there, and then I'll probably be a bit hungover on Sunday morning so a fry up could be the order of the day.

So this week doesn't look too great for my new regime does it?

No, maybe not. Perhaps I'll find something else to wear today. Something that feels a bit looser.

Here we see a clear example of the normally unconscious action of putting on trousers, trigger a conscious thought that leads to an internal dialogue. Very quickly we spot the away from motivation which, in this case, is unsupported by realistic consideration of what specifically would be better than the current situation. There is a desire to do something differently and even a plan for of the practical actions that will be required to achieve a new result, but then there is very little in the way of commitment. Potential success falls at the first hurdle due to the fact that the conservative, short-term side of the inner dialogue comes up with an alternative solution and that alternative will do for now.

As with many examples of inner dialogue, the alternative solution – the one that means we leave things as they are rather than acting on our momentary desire for change – ends up being the most appealing because it means we can avoid having to make too much of an effort beyond our daily routine. We don't experience a different result, but we manage to persuade ourselves that staying as we are isn't too painful after all. The reason we find ourselves following these routines on a regular basis is because we are mostly looking to follow the path of least resistance through life. We're all busy and for many situations where we initially contemplate change, we actually end up quite relieved not to have to make our day busier or more challenging than it already is. But how long does this relief last?

The intention of all behaviour is positive

This is another of the NLP presuppositions. It highlights the fact that we don't deliberately set out to do things that will cause us unhappiness, rather that everything we do is designed to bring us happiness and a positive outcome. The crucial factors that are worth considering within this presupposition are the timing and the quality of the positive experience. When we make our daily decisions, one of the key considerations is always, how long do we have to wait for the pay off from our current behaviour, and how big will the success be?

Managing your weight is a great example of this. In this situation, the inner dialogue is usually between what you've decided you won't allow yourself to eat as part of your overall strategy, and what you think you'd like to eat at any chosen point in the day. For example:

That pasta looks nice but I'm off the carbs at the moment.
Well, surely I can have a little bit.
But if I have a little bit then I'll want more.

A couple of mouthfuls won't hurt.
But then I'll have broken my no carbs plan.
I can get back on the plan later.
Oh go on then.
Doesn't that taste nice?
I'm going to regret this for the rest of the day.

In this example, although it appears at first that we have a conflict between the angel and the devil – the angel advocating sticking with the food plan and the devil suggesting some immediate gratification which would involve behaving contrary to the rules of the plan. In actual fact, the intention of both sides of the dialogue is positive. On the one hand, the experience of eating the pasta would be an immediately enjoyable one, while on the other hand the ability to keep to the rule you've set yourself would be very satisfying when you look back on this moment. One side is arguing for short-term pleasure by eating the pasta, the other side for medium-term pleasure of sticking to your chosen plan.

Enabling your inner dialogue to work for you is all about control and context. It's easy to let your inner dialogue lead you in the right direction if you remember to put every small decision into the context of your overall objectives.

It could be argued that, no matter what the subject of your internal dialogue, many people would veer in the direction of short-term pleasure unless there are some valid options in your head. It's this aspect of our personality that leads us to opt for biscuits instead of fruit, chocolate instead of nuts or a night on the sofa with a glass of wine instead of an evening in the gym. So what's wrong with short-term pleasures?

One difficulty can be that the length of time the short-term pleasure lasts for is far outweighed by the duration of the negative feelings we experience or sometimes impose upon ourselves as a response to that same pleasure.

Insight

Make a list of five recent occasions where you opted for short-term pleasure over medium- to long-term pleasure. Ask yourself, if the same situations arose again, would you make the same decisions?

Our capacity to justify anything that we really want to do is impressive. As is our ability to beat ourselves up at a later date if we don't like the decision we made. The guilt that follows a sweet treat can last for a lot longer than the pleasure of eating the item. It's amazing how emotional we can become, prompted by seemingly the simplest food-related decisions. This need not always be the case, however, and is only really a problem if you lose sight of where each decision is intended to take you. Short-term pleasure is much easier to defer if you know that a longer term and more dramatic or appealing pleasure is possible.

This is where food choices can become tricky for some people. It can require a leap of faith, particularly for those who have had mixed results with weight loss in the past, to convince themselves that deferring the short-term pleasure will bring the long-term pleasure that they're hoping for. What you probably do know all too well though, is the not so positive long-term results of opting for short-term pleasure on a regular basis.

At this point bear in mind your initial objective that you'd like to lose weight and the idea that if you are looking for a different result from that which you have experienced in the past, you will need to begin behaving in a different way. Remember also the notion that there is no failure only feedback.

Focusing on these thoughts should enable you to quickly reduce any negative emotions attached to daily food choices, and step back to allow yourself to assess with a clear head which options will enable you to experience the greatest amount of pleasure over the most lasting period of time.

Adopting this approach can feel very conscious and perhaps even a little forced to begin with. You have to take regular pauses in your daily routine to question the ways you have behaved in the past and make a judgement on what you are going to do for the future. It's precisely because this approach requires a deeper level of conscious engagement that some people are put off adopting it, but be assured that once you have raised the questions about your eating routines that require answers, you will arrive at a situation where you can proceed without the need for any more conscious thought than you give the subject at the moment. You will however be achieving far better results because you will be following new routines that you know, through trial and error, work for you.

Insight

Whenever you adopt a new way of thinking, make a conscious affirmation that you are choosing to behave in this way rather than thinking that behaving in this way implies some kind of compromise in your life. The feeling of positive choice is liberating and empowering. A sense of compromise will limit your enthusiasm and potential results.

Don't tell me what to do

A further issue that causes people hesitation when it comes to making some conscious plans around their strategies for eating and drinking is that they see this process as making 'rules'. The difficulty then for many people is that rules are there to be broken.

Nobody likes being told what to do. You'll notice that's a generalization and clearly there are some people who like being told what to do, but in my experience, when it comes to food and eating habits, not many people enjoy being bossed around (as they may choose to see it). Even those who request, with great conviction, the most detailed food plans and specific instructions tend to go off plan on regular occasions simply because the desire to express some free will, rather than follow a prescribed routine, takes over.

This behaviour is entirely understandable. It's partly due to the fact that many people have deeply engrained beliefs around food, and they also have personal preferences with tastes and textures. Everyone also has a history with food, both personal and cultural, and food can mean many different things to different people, so it can be tricky to encourage anyone to behave in a certain way in relation to their eating. The upshot of this is that if you advise anyone what to eat and drink, the chances are very soon they'll be doing exactly the opposite.

The dislike of rules and regulations can extend to our internal dialogue and, amazingly, even after someone has taken the time to decide on their objectives and plan the appropriate behaviour, the 'devil' is often allowed to triumph in the dialogue. This is simply because they decide that the greatest short-term pleasure of all will be to demonstrate that they are still in charge of their own decision-making, and the desire to override rules and exhibit free will takes precedence over the desire to stick to the rules that they in fact put in place for ourselves.

This is the moment to remember that the intention of all behaviour is still positive. The desire to express free will is positive and has taken over temporarily from the positive desire to eat healthily and achieve a weight loss goal.

At moments like this, referring back to your outcome planning tools will help you assess which of your positively intentioned behaviours will lead to the most desirable results.

It's *your* inner dialogue

Sometimes we are very conscious of the conflicting parts of our inner dialogue and we may even say aloud, 'Part of me knows that I'd feel better if I didn't have this dessert, but part of me really wants to polish the whole lot off.'

Knowing that the intention of all behaviour is positive, aim to reconcile the elements of your inner dialogue by devising win-win solutions for short-, medium- and long-term happiness with all aspects of your dialogue.

The agony of choice?

We are fortunate enough to be faced with choices and options. Let's face it, if you found yourself in too many situations about which you had no choice, you'd soon become pretty aggrieved.

Sometimes having choices can create problems as your inner dialogue struggles to seek out a way of making a decision. Using our inner dialogue to our best advantage is crucial when it comes to effective decision-making.

Given that doing nothing is often not a very productive strategy, particularly when it comes to weight management, if you are really stuck with a decision, sometimes the easiest way to proceed is to simply choose one way to go and get started. You'll get feedback on your progress very quickly that will help you establish if you are heading in the right direction. With this feedback you can refine your approach and then stick with your original decision or try something new. If you find yourself with a recurring internal dialogue, any decision is better than no decision.

For example, if you find yourself overloaded with all the information in the world relating to staying slim, don't waste time wondering which the best weight loss plan to follow is. Get started with one right away and then use the feedback to refine your approach. Similarly with exercise, don't worry about what type of exercise will get you the quickest results, get going with some activity and then adjust the variety of workouts that you do according to the results you are experiencing.

NLP and decision-making

NLP has a selection of techniques that can be employed to investigate the component parts of any choices or decisions you're making, help you maximize the efficiency of your inner dialogues and remove any guesswork involved in decision-making. The first is a process known as chunking.

CHUNKING

No experience or decision exists in isolation but rather every aspect of our thoughts and behaviour is a smaller or greater part of our overall journey through life. Sometimes, and this is certainly true of food and weight management issues, we become preoccupied with the smaller aspects of the situation, with every meal, snack or drink becoming the focal point of all our attention. The danger here is that as the importance of any decision is magnified in our minds, the emotion can intensify until we can no longer experience any sense of perspective on the decision. The process of chunking – moving from general ideas to specifics and vice versa – helps us to make sense of these situations.

When devising a healthy eating routine, many people look at each meal, snack, or drink in isolation. Chunking helps to give perspective and can be used to instil a sense of purpose, often by reminding us of our original objectives. Take snacking for example. Sometimes we are tempted by snack options that might not be the best if we are aiming to achieve our weight loss objectives quickly.

To chunk up, you move from the specific to the general. Ask yourself, 'What is this snack an example of?' Chunking up from snack brings you to food. From food, the next level up is energy. What do you need energy for? To get things done in a day. Why do you need to get things done? To run my life effectively and be happy. In this example, we begin chunking up with the aim of eliciting a higher purpose for your behaviour. As you begin to ask these higher purpose questions, you may see your initial snack temptation in a new light.

For example, if you were thinking about having a snack and fancied a muffin, how do you feel about it in relation to your higher purpose? If your objective is to be happy, what part does eating a muffin play in making you happy? How long will the happiness of eating the muffin last? How long will the benefits of not eating the muffin last? Are there alternatives you can snack on that will be more likely to make you happy in the short, medium and long-term?

Chunking down from the term 'snack' can also help provide alternative options. A question that helps you to chunk down in this example is, 'If I think of a snack, what would be an example of a snack I could have now?' The reply in this case could be cakes, muffins, biscuits, fruit, nuts, yoghurt, or crudités. Within each of these categories you will immediately see a variety of options.

At this point, it might be a good idea to make a distinction between healthy snacks or 'treat' snacks. Healthy snacks are those you'd be happy to eat at any time. Treat snacks are those that can be consumed in moderation. Your specific food plan will eventually show you the right level of moderation for you. As time progresses, you should also aim to create a list of options at this level that is as varied as possible in order that you have choices you can make for any given circumstances. This will enable you to always stick to your plan and achieve your objectives without ever needing to think too much about what the possibilities are for each snack.

Insight
Dividing food into categories such as healthy snacks and treat snacks is not to imply that some foods are 'good' while others are 'bad'. It merely serves to help with planning your expectations when it comes to quantity and frequency of different options in your schedule.

Provided you keep your higher purpose in mind and do some research to develop a list of choices and options that will help you achieve this higher purpose, you need not agonize over every food decision that you are faced with each day. You can see very clearly from this example that if you chunk from snacks to food to energy,

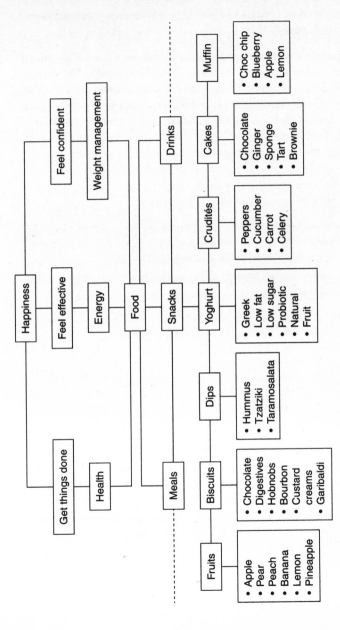

Figure 8.1 Chunking a food tree.

you can quickly contextualize your snack options by asking yourself 'Which of these options will provide me with energy and which will rob me of energy?'

Chunking up or down is the process of moving from the specific to the general, or vice versa. You will know from personal experience that there are individuals who prefer to work with detail and others who prefer just the headlines, and who feel overwhelmed when you begin to provide them with any kind of detail. Having clarity on which mode of operating you prefer will help you with your weight loss objectives. If you are someone who likes to know strategy and headlines, maintaining clear images in your mind as to what your objectives are and why they matter can often be enough to dictate your daily behaviour and keep you on track.

If you are a details person you may wish to put together a lengthy step-by-step plan to take you through each day from now until the point in the future that you know you will have achieved your goal. Think about it now, from your previous experiences, which approach suits you best?

Make sure your current approach is the right one for you. If you are someone who prefers the overview, try not to get bogged down with detail or you'll lose sight of why you set your objectives in the first place. If you are a details person, remember to include regular planning and updating of your approach to ensure you're always heading in the right direction and then design the finer points of the routine that will get you to your goal as quickly as possible.

PARTS INTEGRATION AND DECISION-MAKING

The second technique to help maximize the efficiency of your inner dialogue is known as parts integration. It's a process that allows you to unite two seemingly opposing parts of your personality and your inner dialogue, and reconcile them so that you can move forwards more effectively towards your objective. This technique can provide a very effective solution to the daily dilemmas relating to short, medium or long-term pleasure. If you ever find yourself thinking things along the lines of, 'There's a part of me that would love to stick with this healthy eating routine, but there's also a part of me that would really enjoy being able to forget the whole thing,' then this is a technique for you.

As with most NLP techniques there is a specific system to follow to make this process the most effective. Here's how it goes.

1 **Separate the parts**
   Clearly identify and separate the parts in conflict. To continue with our snacking example from above, it could be that one part of you would like the pleasure of a piece of cake now while the other part of you wants to stick to your plan of eating cake only once a week.

2 **Get a clear representation of each part**
   It can help when there are two parts of a dilemma, to place one part in the palm of each hand. Get representations of each part using visual, kinaesthetic and auditory prompts. What does each part look like, how do they feel? What do they sound like? What's the history of each part? Think about why you want the cake and place all the sights, sounds, feelings tastes and smells associated with eating cake in one hand. Think about why you want to avoid the cake and put all the sights, sounds, feelings, tastes and smells associated with not eating cake in the other hand.

3 **Find out the intention of each part**
   Chunk up until you are able to find a common positive intention for the two parts. Keep in mind that the intention of all behaviour is positive and that both parts have your best interests at heart, in some way. One part is thinking of your short-term pleasure while the other part is focused on your longer-term pleasure. You can use this information to begin negotiating between the two parts in the same way as you would witness a negotiation between two people.

4 **Establish negotiating points**
   Find out what resources each part has that would help the other realize its concern. Where are the points of agreement? What does each part want from the other to be satisfied? It soon becomes obvious that the act of conflict prevents each part from achieving its desired end.

5 **Ask each part if it is willing to integrate with the other to solve their shared problems**
   It's useful here to have a physical representation of what's going on mentally, so if you have placed the two parts in the palms of your hands, physically push them together. Sometimes as you are

negotiating with the two parts, you suddenly realize they have moved closer together unconsciously. Now create the picture, sounds, feelings, smells and tastes associated with the new, integrated part, and absorb it into yourself at the pace that feels right for you.

Take your time here as this new part enables you to review past events and experiences through the lens of your new understanding. Don't be concerned if during your parts integration or negotiation, other arguments come to mind. This is to be expected – if your inner conflict is deep seated, both sides of the argument will have built up plenty of ammunition over the years – and if you allow different voices to join the negotiation, accessing the higher purpose for each of them, you'll eventually arrive at the most thorough resolution.

Neither should you be concerned if you sense elements of the same conflict arising within you in the future. This is natural and is merely the way in which your mind regularly reviews whether or not the conclusions you came to during the integration are still the right ones. You should be in the habit of regularly reviewing all thoughts, behaviours and attitudes to guarantee that your current state of mind in relation to your objectives is the correct one for success. Keeping your higher purpose in mind, you can embrace many aspects of your inner dialogue and keep your mind open to new ideas, thoughts and experiences to be discussed and channelled for your future success.

A clear path forwards

These techniques are designed to help you position your mind for success and deal with any internal conflicts that could slow your progress. Removing barriers to success is fundamental to any project so, if you're ever struggling to find an immediate solution, ask yourself, 'What's stopping me from making progress here?' and then apply some of the techniques you've learned so far.

Chapter 9 contains a selection of further techniques that will ensure you're never stuck for ideas on how to tackle your weight management and stay slim for good.

Inner dialogue

Use every conversation in your head to your advantage.

Presupposition: the intention of all behaviour is positive

A useful thought to bear in mind when considering your own behaviour and the behaviour of others.

Chunking

Ensure positive decision-making by examining the bigger picture as well as the finer details of every situation.

Parts integration

Resolve internal conflict quickly and easily; make decisions and proceed effectively.

10 THINGS TO REMEMBER

1 How you choose to communicate with yourself is as important as how you communicate with others.

2 Listen to the voices in your head.

3 Pay attention to the questions you ask yourself and challenge the assertions you make.

4 Be specific with the dialogue inside your head. Seek answers and solutions and don't leave questions hanging open-ended.

5 Remember, the intention of all behaviour is positive. Analyse everything you and others do until you can isolate the positive intention. Then establish how to fulfil the positive intention without any negative consequences.

6 Think 'choices' rather than 'obligation'. You are in charge of your own destiny at all times. Remember this.

7 Chunk up. You can make decision-making easier by assessing each decision in the context of your higher purpose or life mission.

8 Chunk down. You can increase your options in any situation by examining the details of your choices.

9 When making decisions, consider balance over the long term. This can ease perceived pressure on the short and medium term.

10 Seek win–win situations. Even in what seems to be the most extreme internal conflict, there will be common ground between the parts in conflict. Establishing what this is will help you move forward.

9

More NLP techniques to help you stay slim for good

In this chapter you will learn:
- *a quick technique to end negative behaviours and turn them into positives*
- *how to use your time line to determine your weight management future*
- *how to live with great weight management results, starting right now.*

Six-step reframing

A similar process to parts integration, known as six-step reframing, can be used to address any aspect of your behaviour that you feel hinders your progress towards your weight loss goal. Many NLP practitioners use the technique of parts integration rather than the six step reframing process, but in a world where the person with the greatest flexibility will control the system, it's useful to have knowledge of as many techniques as possible.

The behaviour to be changed could be unconscious or conscious, but will not always lead to an internal dialogue conflict. It could simply be something that you know you do regularly but you'd rather this behaviour was no longer a part of your life. It could be that you feel you drink too many fizzy drinks, you snack on foods that prevent you from reaching your objectives quickly, or you eat too much at mealtimes.

The process of reframing involves separating the positive intention of the behaviour – and you'll remember that the intention of all behaviour is positive – from the aspect of the behaviour that causes you stress or anxiety. This will enable you to achieve the positive intention of the behaviour without any negative consequences. Here's how it works.

1. Relax and focus on the behaviour you'd like to change.
2. Establish communication with the part of you responsible for the behaviour you'd like to change. Ask this part to give you a signal if it is willing to communicate with you. Notice any internal sounds, images or feelings.
3. When you have a clear signal, you must ask the part to reveal the positive intention behind the behaviour you'd like to change.
4. Ask the part of you responsible for creative behaviour to suggest at least three alternative ways to achieve the same positive intention as the behaviour that you'd like to change.
5. Ask the part responsible for the behaviour you'd like to change if it is willing to use any of the alternative choices in the near future. If you sense there is some barrier to using the alternative choices for the moment, ask the part when it will be ready to begin using some of the alternatives. Use the creative part of you to suggest other alternatives that could be implemented for a limited period to begin with.
6. Check that the part of you responsible for the behaviour is happy to proceed without reservation with the agreed alternative behaviour. If you sense some hesitation, return to step three and repeat the process, adding further options on new behaviour. Continue the process until you feel confident that the new behaviour will replace the old behaviour from this moment onwards.

Here's how the process could run when it comes to staying slim for good.

The behaviour you want to change is to stop snacking on sugary food when you are bored.

You may notice that the part responsible for this behaviour resides in your stomach, your chest or in your head.

The positive intention behind this behaviour is to alleviate boredom and give you a lift when you feel your mood drop.

Three alternative ways to give you a lift could be to make a telephone call, spend a little time doing something you enjoy, perhaps a hobby or social networking, or change your physical environment by going for a walk.

If you're not completely convinced that these three alternatives will work, others could be that you distract yourself by reading a book or a magazine, or you could snack but select alternatives to the sugary options that you are trying to avoid.

The process is complete when you are convinced that the next time you feel bored you'll gravitate towards one of these suggested alternative behaviours and won't be tempted to snack on sugary foods.

Once again, this process illustrates the notion that when it comes to the thoughts and behaviours that achieve success with weight loss, context and balance are key, and that many of our behaviours that are positive in intention only become negative in excess. Fortunately there is always an alternative behaviour or, in many cases, a moderation of our current behaviour to strike the right balance between achieving the positive intention of all behaviour, without the negative consequence.

To successfully stay slim for good, you don't have to change everything or give up everything. You simply need to determine the right balance of all your behaviours.

This reminds us also that there is no such thing as a bad food, merely inappropriate quantities or timing of these foods. An additional guideline worth remembering is that just because some amount of various foods or drinks is good, this doesn't necessarily mean that more is better. Think about caffeine, alcohol, chocolate, cakes and biscuits. All can have their place in the schedule that brings you success with your weight management objectives, but all must be consumed in the correct quantities and with appropriate frequency. With the right balance of every behaviour, you can benefit from the positive intention without tipping over into negative consequences or repercussions. All you need to do is experiment until you find the right balance and then stick to this consistently.

Insight

When you've established the balance that's right for you, behave consistently with this balance. Do not be tempted to have 'just one more' or 'just a little bit extra', 'just this once'. Stick with what you know works and enjoy the results, not the 'extras'.

Time lines

You'll notice that, once again, a key factor in applying NLP techniques to help you achieve your objectives centres around making sure that your thoughts and attitudes are up to date and consistent with what you are trying to achieve. To assist with this process yet further, NLP has a technique specifically designed to help you work with your past, present and future more easily and to assist you in managing your state of mind at all times.

We're all aware of our past, we're living in the present and, hopefully we all believe that we'll have a successful future. Limitations to success can arise if you feel that you were not, or are not, in control of any, or all, of these parts of your life, also known as your time line. The technique known as time line therapy will help you gain control and perspective in all areas of your past, present and future.

Time line therapy suggests that you view your journey through life as a physical line running through your body with the past extending off in one direction and the future extending in another direction. Your body marks the point on your time line where you are now – the present. The idea behind this thinking is that if you can place events of the past and present in a physical space, this enables you to 'visit' events of the future or revisit events of the past. By moving along your time line in this way, you can both examine events of the past and reframe them if necessary and you can plan events of the future in greater detail which will, in turn, make your anticipated outcome more likely. Working with your past and future in this way helps you make sense of the present and what's happening in your life right now.

As we've discussed earlier in the book, beliefs and values are formed in response to specific events and interaction with those around us, and they help us make sense of our daily lives. We've looked at how to update limiting beliefs and how to spring clean your beliefs so they are consistent with what you would currently like to achieve.

For some deeply held beliefs, you may need some extra help in bringing them up to date and this is where working with your time line is helpful. The technique enables you to revisit the moments in the past when these beliefs were formed and, with the knowledge that the intention of all behaviour is positive, you can understand why you might cling to these beliefs in the present.

Here's an extreme example to illustrate the point. Imagine an individual who thinks at some stage of their life that they want to make sure they never become overweight. This notion has a positive intention, which is that they want to ensure they never feel physically unwell, and that they always want to look their best and feel confident and happy in their own skin.

At some point, this initial thought, along with its positive intention, turns into a deeply held belief that being overweight is a terrible thing, and that because eating too much is the behaviour most likely to lead to you becoming overweight, and that therefore food is bad. This belief leads the individual to eat less food with the result that they remain slim and their belief becomes reinforced week after week until they begin to associate eating less with becoming thinner, and being thinner as a measure of greater success in their ability to avoid becoming overweight. At the very extreme end of this process, there is a danger this person can begin to avoid eating at all costs. In this case, what was originally a positive thought – to be vigilant about your body weight to remain healthy and happy – has become something that is actually physically harmful, and is at the same time unlikely to lead to happiness.

Time line therapy can help to investigate many of our current beliefs and behaviours by revisiting the moment when these beliefs were originally formed and analysing the results of these beliefs, their associated behaviours and the ways in which some positive intentions and behaviours can become confused over time. By using time line therapy, we can update beliefs and revise behaviours based on how these past behaviours have shaped our present and are likely to shape our future. Here's how to use time line therapy to your advantage.

ELICITING YOUR TIME LINE

Think of events in the past. Where do you see them in physical space? Are they in front of you, behind you or stretching off to the side in one direction or the other? Now think of something that you'll be doing in the future. What position do these tasks inhabit? Where are they in relation to the memories of the past?

At this point, it may be useful to explain that there are two distinct ways in which people organize time. There are some exceptions, but generally these are the ways in which the majority of people arrange their time line.

If when you think of the past, you position events to your left or slightly in front of you, and when you think of the future, you position events to your right or slightly in front of you in a different direction to the past, you have a preference for organizing time in a way that's known as 'through time'.

If when you think of the past, you position events behind you and when you think of the future, you position events in front of you, you have a preference for organizing time in a way that's known as 'in time'.

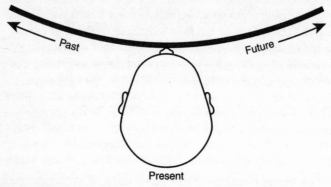

Figure 9.1 'Through time' time line.

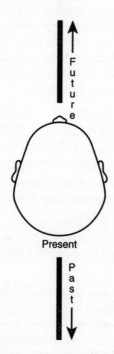

Figure 9.2 'In time' time line.

ORGANIZING TIME AND MANAGING WEIGHT

There are a number of characteristics associated with the ways in which people organize time. Knowledge of these characteristics can be very helpful when examining your past behaviours relating to managing your weight and considering how you can modify your current behaviour to affect the future and achieve new results.

Living through time

'Through time' people like to plan; they are very organized and don't like to repeat behaviours they perceive to be mistakes. Aspects of a through time personality that are beneficial to staying slim are: the ability to sit down and plan in great detail what needs to happen to achieve their goals. Aspects of a through time personality that can hinder staying slim are: inflexibility if the plan doesn't run smoothly, a tendency to be hard on oneself if things don't work out and a difficulty in maintaining the 'no failure, only feedback' perspective, which can result in a loss of motivation.

Living in time

'In time' people do not particularly like to plan; they like to live for the moment. They're not big fans of the clock. They appear to be more spontaneous than through time people, and tend to be focused on doing what they enjoy at any given time, rather than following a specific schedule of events. Whereas through time people are usually on time or early for appointments, in time people are more likely to be late, although they often don't consider themselves to be late. Their feeling is that as long as they arrive when they are ready, that moment is the beginning of the appointment.

Aspects of an in time person that are beneficial to staying slim forever are: flexibility of behaviour and a willingness to try new options at any given moment. Aspects of an in time personality that can hinder staying slim are: the tendency to focus on short-term rather than medium- or long-term results and an inability to put current behaviours into the context of the bigger picture results.

Insight

Consider the way in which you organize time and examine how you can approach things differently in the future to achieve the weight loss results you are looking for. You may wish to be a bit more organized. Or you may decide that a little more flexibility in your behaviour would be beneficial. You may decide you need to plan your actions in more detail and be more disciplined, or you may perceive that you need to go with the flow a little more and not be so self-critical.

TIME LINES AND BELIEF CHANGE

Regardless of how you organize time, you can make good use of your time line to work on changing any of your beliefs that may have become detrimental to staying slim for good. The good news is this is quite a simple process.

1 Highlight the behaviour that you think needs updating.
2 Imagine hovering above your time line and travelling into the past to the event where you first formed the belief that ultimately led to the behaviour that you think now needs updating.
3 Ask yourself, what specifically was the positive intention of forming this belief? You may need to spend a few moments running through some options here and maybe chunking up to establish the highest priority positive intention at the time.
4 Hover above your time line and return towards the present, examining incidences of when this belief and its associated behaviour served you well and when this belief and its associated behaviour tipped the balance from doing you good to doing you harm. For each of these instances, come up with some suggestions on what behaviour would have been more appropriate at the time.
5 Return to the present. You are now armed with an understanding of the positive intention of your belief and a selection of options for alternative behaviours that would achieve the same positive intention. Consider how this new knowledge will affect your current frame of mind. You will feel upbeat, motivated and in control.
6 Hover above your time line and travel to the future, to a time when you think your old belief and associated behaviour would have dictated your results in this situation, and imagine instead exercising one of your alternative behaviours. Imagine all the options of how this may lead to different outcomes.

FORWARD PLAN SUCCESSFUL BEHAVIOUR CHANGE

If you're struggling with the notion of behaving differently at some stage in the near future, remove any limitations in time and then travel further forwards to the point at which you are able to look back towards the present and know that you have successfully behaved in the way that you are finding difficult to implement at the moment.

This sounds complicated but, if you think about it, most behaviours, particularly those we are already a little unhappy with, have an expiry date on them. A time by which we know we'll have changed these behaviours – even highly addictive habits such as smoking, for example. When asked about their habit, many smokers express the desire to give up at some stage. Some would like to give up now, others at some point in the future. To bring clarity to the time at which they will give up, you can ask a smoker to think forwards in time as far as is necessary to visualize the desired result. Will they still be a smoker in a week, a month, a year, two years, five years, ten years, fifteen years? At some point along this time line they'll respond with, 'oh no, I definitely won't be smoking in x years time. I'll have given up by then.'

Think about your food routine and your weight management in the same way. At what point in your future do you make the transition from dieting and battling with your weight to following a healthy eating pattern that brings you consistent weight management results? How far along your timeline do you need to travel in the future to the point at which you will look back on dieting from a position of success? When you will have mastered healthy eating once and for all? If you are currently persisting with trying different approaches to healthy eating, you must be convinced that this moment will arrive at some point in your future.

As you visualize this time, associate into it and alter the submodalities of the moment. Turn up the brightness, the volume, increase the power of the positive feelings you experience when you reach this time. Keep working on the moment until you make it as exciting as you can. If you can get this excited about achieving these feelings in the future, why wait to experience them? Is there anything preventing you from taking action to achieve success with healthy eating right now? When you feel as positive as you can about your imagined future, hover above your time line, move back to the present and reassess your current objectives through this lens of positive emotion. You'll find that this process greatly increases your desire to behave in the way that will produce these emotions again, sooner rather than later.

Working with your time line helps both to reinterpret the past in a positive way and to remove some of the uncertainties of the future. With regular practise, you will become accustomed to the habit of learning from the past to optimize the present and determine your future, without it feeling like such a conscious process.

Utilizing your full personal resources

As you know, NLP works both with your conscious mind and your unconscious mind, and working with your time line is a further example of how you can utilize your full mental capacity to increase your chances of personal success. Regular conscious interaction with your time line will ensure that your unconscious mind is always using the learning of the past and the present to help you achieve the greatest success for the future.

Occasionally it is precisely the strength of the desire to achieve something that can lead to a difficulty in committing to it fully and you may experience a situation where, because your objective is so important, you feel almost afraid of it and this can lead to hesitation in your behaviour. Simply due to the fact that there is so much to gain and the results are so desirable, there may be a part of you that hesitates because you fear that you may not be successful in your outcome, and if you're not successful, this can have a negative impact on your self confidence.

We've discussed how NLP techniques can be employed to clear out any thoughts that may hinder your success, integrate parts that may be in conflict, and help you position your attitudes and behaviour to ensure that you can take advantage of all opportunities to make your journey to success quicker and easier.

In some cases, a hint of reservation may still remain simply because you are entering uncharted water. If you've never achieved the specific result you're setting out for, you may still experience a very small voice in your head casting slight doubt over your chances of success. If you find yourself in this situation, don't worry. NLP has a solution for this too.

ACT AS IF

I'm sure you will have come across the phrase 'fake it until you make it'. It was designed for exactly this situation and it can be a very useful skill. Employing it means that, even though you may not be entirely convinced that the way in which you are behaving feels right or will lead you to your desired outcome, simply acting as if you are the person you'd like to become, or behaving as though you have already achieved the goals that you'd like to achieve, is often the final part of the jigsaw that allows all the other pieces to fall into place.

The key to quick success with many objectives is confidence, and confidence often comes simply from experience. The danger here is if you think you will become confident in doing something after you've done it a few times, how will you ever do it for the first time? If you wait until you feel you have the confidence to do something, you could be waiting for a long time.

As ever, NLP takes an alternative view of the situation and suggests that if you can bring yourself to take a leap of faith and begin taking action first, the confidence in these actions will follow very quickly. Public speaking is a good example of this principle in action. Many people don't like the idea of public speaking, in fact in some studies the fear of public speaking is often reported to be greater than the fear of dying. Chances are, though, if you were to deliver the same presentation or speech a number of times, you would begin to feel more comfortable with doing it. Who knows, you may even enjoy it.

Regardless of how you feel delivering your presentation, your audience won't have any idea how many times you've done the presentation before, how confident you are or how good you are. So just pretend that your first audience is your fiftieth and that you step up to your first presentation feeling full of confidence and assured in your own ability. Providing you've done your research and preparation thoroughly, approaching your presentation acting as if you're brimming with confidence will minimize your anxiety and maximize your success on the day.

Acting 'as if' helps speed results with weight loss dramatically. Many people embark on a weight loss project with some good ideas of what life will be like when they have achieved their objectives. If you do your homework properly, employing the relevant NLP techniques, you'll have a very clear visualization of what your future holds and will be hugely motivated to manoeuvre yourself towards this situation swiftly. So, if you're able to imagine living with so many benefits brought into your life by achieving your goal in the future, why wait to experience those benefits? Why not start acting as if you are in this position right now?

If you think losing weight will make you confident, act as if you are already oozing with confidence. If you think losing weight will make you a more friendly person, start acting as if you are already a friendly person. If you think achieving and maintaining your target weight will make you happy and fulfilled, begin acting like a happy and fulfilled person right away.

The benefits of acting as if are simple:

▶ It helps build confidence.
▶ It helps you learn more about the key information you need to achieve sustained success with your objectives. It's one thing to imagine and anticipate what you might need to know, another thing to gather real life information that you can act upon quickly.
▶ It keeps you on track with the behaviours that will hasten your positive outcome. The more you try out and get use to living with the positive experiences associated with your outcome, the more likely you are to stick with the behaviours that will ensure this outcome becomes an ongoing reality sooner rather than later.

The final benefit of acting as if is that by filling your head with new thoughts, specifically the thoughts of someone who has become the person they'd like to be, and left behind the person they felt they had outgrown, you'll notice that you concern yourself less with the thoughts that held you back in your quest for weight loss and focus much more on positive thoughts that speed you on your way to long-term success. There's no motivation like a bit of progress, and acting as if enables you to take a big step forwards mentally which will be quickly followed by tangible, physical changes.

Insight
When it comes to acting as if, build your confidence gradually by changing your behaviour in subtle ways to begin with, and then move on to increase the number of environments in which you test out your new behaviour.

Modelling

When I think back to when I was learning to drive, I distinctly recall feeling quite apprehensive about the whole idea. If I think about it too vividly, I can actually feel some of the anxiety that I experienced then, building up inside my stomach. Part of the anxiety was due to the fact that being able to drive was an objective that really mattered to me. I was desperate to get my driving licence and I really wanted to pass my test first time. I knew at the time that it was good to be a little nervous as this would help me engage in learning the skills I needed but I also remember thinking that if I worried too much about the whole process it probably wouldn't help. So I thought about how I could make the whole experience a little less daunting.

I decided to try to diminish my anxiety at learning to drive by thinking about the enormous number of people who had already managed to do it. I remember repeatedly looking around at other drivers thinking if they can all do this, so can I. If they can learn the skills and pass the driving test, there's no reason why I shouldn't be able to do it. I started observing other drivers, looking at their faces, their demeanour and their style of driving, imagining what they were thinking as they drove around. I even went as far as watching people walking down the street and imagining what kind of a driver they would be when they got behind the wheel of a car.

I found these thoughts very comforting. After all, those other drivers were only human. They had the same type of mind and body as I had, and I had the ability to learn this skill just as they had. I know now that one of the presuppositions of NLP is that 'if one person can do something, anyone can learn to do it', and this is one of the reasons why I find NLP so useful – it has the ability to very succinctly take thoughts that have occurred to you at one time or another and condense these into useful phrases, techniques and guidelines to live your life by. And it's all rooted in common sense.

The process of using others as inspiration for your undertakings or 'copying' the success of others is called modelling and it's something you will have done, consciously or unconsciously, many times in your life. You do it unconsciously when you're younger as you absorb the behaviour and values of family and friends, and you do it more consciously when you're older as you model the fashions, attitudes ideas and strategies of friends, colleagues and those in the media.

Modelling is useful for weight management. After all, what is a diet plan but a model of a strategy that has been published by someone whose opinion and achievements we admire and would like to emulate?

Just like outcome planning, modelling is most successful when you get really specific and cater for the full range of representational systems. Think about your weight loss role models as you apply the following elements of modelling.

VISUAL MODELLING

Model those who you would like to emulate by watching how they behave. This includes how they behave in as many different circumstances as possible and over as long a time frame as possible. The more aspects of successful behaviour you are witness to, the easier it is to emulate the results these behaviours produce.

AUDITORY MODELLING

Model those you admire by asking them how they achieve their success. Find an opportunity to speak with them and run through a sequence of prepared questions that will help you highlight their strategies and attitudes. If your role models are in the public eye, you probably won't be able to speak with them directly but you can research as many interviews with them as possible and cross reference what you read in different publications and on websites until you can put together consistent elements of their thoughts and behaviours.

KINAESTHETIC MODELLING

Try on different elements of your role models' behaviour and see how you feel about them. Get a sense of the emotions you'll experience by adopting elements of the behaviours of others. Once you're comfortable with how the behaviours feel, you can try them out in reality and see what works for you.

SPREAD YOUR MODELLING NET AS WIDE AS POSSIBLE

Your success with your outcome will depend on your flexibility with your role models. Take the best bits of a variety of other people's approaches, the sections of their strategies that most appeal to you and your specific situation, and put together the specific approach that works for you.

The advantage of modelling is that it means you don't have to break new ground with everything you think you need to learn to make your outcome a reality. Borrowing success from other people is a clever way to save yourself time and effort, and the benefit of the approach is that there is almost always someone out there who has already completed what you want to achieve. Fast track your route to success by asking them how they did it. Remember also there is no limit to modelling. There will always be a great supply of subjects to model and each of the strategies you learn from others can be employed in a variety of different situations at any stage in your future.

CHOOSE YOUR FRIENDS WISELY

Like all NLP skills, modelling becomes easier as you practise it, and also when you increase your exposure to a greater number of people acting in the way that you find motivating and achieving the kind of results that you find inspiring. This means that it's wise to spend as much time as you can with people who behave how you'd like to behave. Surround yourself with people who you can learn from and your quest for success will be much easier.

Be aware also that surrounding yourself with too many people who are currently facing the same issues and challenges as you can lead to stalled progress or even regression. Try if you can to associate with people who are ahead of you on the journey for results, rather than spending too much time with those at the same stage of progress or who may even be behind you in their progress. It's better to be with people you admire and who will lift you up to their level than spend too much time with those you don't admire or who could drag you down to their level. In the words of a poster I once saw, 'It's hard to soar with eagles when you're surrounded by turkeys!' Make sure you associate with more eagles than turkeys.

Don't drive with the brakes on
Consider groups of friends or work colleagues up and down the country. There are some that continually discuss their quest for weight loss, the latest diet or routine they are on, their constant frustrations with the barriers they face or their inconsistent results, and they regularly derail each other with the choices they make or encourage others to make by joining them.

Jump on the coat-tails of those who succeed
There are also many groups that motivate each other with discussions and behaviours that are consistent with their individual and shared weight loss objective. They share ideas and success strategies leading to faster progress for each member of the group.

How's your circle of influence?
Think about the people you work with and associate with. Does their behaviour and their actions help you in your weight loss goals?

Can you learn from them? Can you model their strategies and apply them to your own situation? Make sure that you spend as much time as possible in environments full of people who support your objectives and who inspire you to great things.

Model your own success

An additional element to modelling is that the benefits of the technique are not limited to modelling other people. You can build confidence in your abilities by modelling your own successes of the past. If you take the time to think about it, you will be able to recall many examples when you successfully achieved something you set out to do. It doesn't matter what the experience relates to, what matters is that you can use these experiences to conjure up the thoughts and feelings associated with your most successful state of being.

WHAT HAVE YOU DONE WELL IN THE PAST?

Take a moment now to think about a time when you were aware of a great sense of achievement, fulfilment, satisfaction and triumph. Where were you when you experienced these feelings? What had you achieved? What led you to this success? Was it easy or hard to achieve? Did you feel as though you had to earn your success? Did you achieve success by yourself or with the help of others?

As you think about this moment, what can you see? What can you hear? What specific feelings are you experiencing? Are there any smells or tastes associated with these memories?

The more detail you can add to the recollection, the easier it will be to consider how you achieved this success and to then copy the methods you used and apply them to any current challenges you are facing. Thinking about this experience and others that are similar, I'm sure you'll notice some familiar concepts, many of which you may have been unaware of previously but you'll now recognize as key NLP components in your success. It's likely that to achieve this success you would have had a clear plan, a well-formed outcome including resources, deadlines and all the imagined benefits of achieving this goal. It's also likely that you would have engaged your conscious mind in helping you to achieve your success as well as using your unconscious mind throughout the process.

As you think through the details of your previous successes, write down all the elements of your approach that you can utilize now to help with your weight management objectives.

Now follow the same process for as many other examples as you can think of when you have been successful in the past. The more examples you can think of, the easier it will become for you to highlight your modus operandi – the key ingredients and strategies that lead you to successful behaviour – and you will then be able to apply these strategies to future challenges.

WHAT DO YOU DO WELL NOW?

When modelling yourself, consider also which areas of your current routine are successful. There will be many things you do, probably without thinking too much about them, where you achieve quick and efficient success. It is precisely because you do these things without thinking and can achieve success in these areas unconsciously that you can easily overlook the skills that you employ to achieve this success. Bring these strategies into your conscious mind and analyse which elements of these strategies you can draw across and apply to your weight loss objectives. Think about the following questions:

- ▶ In which areas of your life do you find success easy?
- ▶ How do you achieve this success?
- ▶ How do you organize these projects/tasks?
- ▶ What's your mindset when you approach these projects/tasks?
- ▶ What techniques do you utilize for these projects/tasks?
- ▶ What resources do you tap into for these projects/tasks?

Sum up the secret of your success in these areas in a maximum of five words.

Now think about how you can apply the above information to your weight loss objectives. For example, if you have a successful and enjoyable social life, begin to analyse how you achieve success in this area so you can adapt the same approach to weight management.

In which areas of your life do you find success easy?
I have a really good social life.

How do you achieve this success?
I spend quality time with the people that matter to me.

How do you organize these projects/tasks?
I make a point of seeing people regularly and speaking to them between social events.

What's your mindset when you approach these projects/tasks?
I look forward to making these arrangements because I know I'll have a good time.

What techniques do you utilize for these projects/tasks?
I check my mental social calendar every day so I know what's coming up and I update my paper diary every couple of days. I get in touch with my friends at least once a week and arrange to meet whenever possible.

What resources do you tap into for these projects/tasks?
I need to be organized with my commitments at home and I need the support of my partner for child care when appropriate. I need to be efficient with delegation at work to ensure I have time for my social engagements.

Sum up the secret of your success in these areas in a maximum of five words:
time management; planning; enjoyment; balance.

TRANSFERABLE SKILLS

The strategies employed for success in this area are simple and they work because the upside of making them work is compelling enough. Run through this exercise for as many areas of life in which you feel you are successful, and compile a list of your own success strategies that you can model and apply to help with your weight loss. Title the list 'How I make myself successful: secrets of success keywords'.

Pay particular attention to the keywords that sum up the secret of your success in a variety of areas. Compile a list of all the keywords and then make sure you can apply them all to your weight management objectives.

The right mindset for success

Recalling previous successful experiences is good for the spirit. In fact, taking time to let any positive thoughts run through your mind is a valuable experience and can quickly alter your view of what's going on around you. Most people would agree that your mood of the moment can make an enormous difference to how well you get on with the projects you are working on and the people you are interacting with. How often have you found yourself struggling with an idea, only to return to it later in a better frame of mind and find a solution right away? How many times have you found other people irritating, only to look back on the meeting later and realize that your irritation was attributable to the fact that something else had put you in a bad mood?

So, to have control over our frame of mind at any given point is a great asset in determining the success and enjoyment of our day-to-day lives. Taking time in your day to focus on the positive is always helpful for boosting your mood and your access to your inner resources. For times when you really need a burst of positive energy, there's an NLP technique that you can use. It's called anchoring.

PACK UP POSITIVE EMOTIONS

Anchoring enables you to 'store' your most positive feelings and emotions and then tap into them when you need them most. In your quest for your ideal healthy eating routine, you may be challenged by other people or by your own thoughts and doubts, so to be able to tap into your most resourceful state when you need it can prove invaluable. The technique boosts your resilience to all challenges you may face along the way and works very simply by associating or 'anchoring' a physical gesture with your most positive state of mind. Here's how it works.

1 Think of a time when you felt positive and successful.
2 Associate yourself into this experience and acknowledge the emotions that were present at the time.
3 Grow these emotions by turning up the submodalities of your experience. Make it brighter, clearer, louder, more intense.
4 Continue growing the intensity of the experience in your head until you can experience a powerful representation of the physical feelings you had at the time. This is likely to manifest itself as a feeling of excitement, butterflies in the stomach and shortness of breath.
5 As you feel the experience build to the peak of its intensity, 'anchor' the feelings with a physical gesture. This gesture should be something you can replicate subtly when you want to experience your positive state, but not a physical movement that you do on a regular basis. Something like pressing your thumb and little finger together or pressing your ring finger firmly into the side of your leg will work well.

Having worked through the process of anchoring, you will be able to instantly reach your peak state by activating your physical gesture when you need it. You can also grow the effectiveness of the technique by 'stacking' other positive experiences and feelings on top of the same physical anchor. The more positive experiences you have stacked on top of each other, the more intense the positive feelings will be when you activate your physical trigger.

NLP tools to help you stay slim for good

Six-step reframing

Use this further method to refine your attitude for success.

Time line therapy

Learn from the past, optimize the present, determine your future.

Act as if

Begin success behaviours right now.

Modelling

Learn from the success of others and transfer your own success skills to all areas of your life.

Anchoring

Lock in your most powerful, positive mindset.

10 THINGS TO REMEMBER

1   The more NLP techniques you have at your disposal, the greater your flexibility to take control in any circumstance.

2   No experience in the past is entirely negative. There is a lesson in every event that can be used for the future.

3   Check in with yourself every day to ensure that your current thoughts and behaviours are consistent with the results you are trying to achieve.

4   Plant positive outcomes in your future timeline to enable your unconscious mind to be working towards these outcomes at all times.

5   Adopt the attitudes and behaviours of success immediately.

6   Remain alert to people that you can model every day.

7   Check that the company you keep helps you to progress your weight loss objectives.

8   Always be aware of your own successful strategies, attitudes and communication skills in order that you can utilize these in all areas of your life.

9   Take time to acknowledge and fully engage with the feelings of success. Anchor positive sensations and thoughts for use in the future.

10 Practise these techniques regularly. The more you practise, the sooner the techniques can become unconscious and these methods of engaging with events at a deeper level will become second nature.

10

Bullet-proof weight management: how to guarantee you stay slim for good

In this chapter you will learn:
- *the four stages of the learning process that will ensure ongoing success*
- *how a variety of techniques can be applied to real-life situations*
- *suggested NLP routes to long-term success with staying slim.*

Along the path to staying slim forever there will be challenges. When you feel confident that the strategies you have developed are able to withstand whatever obstacles you come across, you can safely say that when it comes to this particular area of your life, you are bullet-proof.

To be bullet-proof when it comes to your healthy eating and weight management plan means that you are following the routines that work for you without having to think about your every decision. Mastering your food routine is a very liberating experience because at this point you will have learned to live a life where you no longer question what you eat, when you eat it, and how you feel about each meal and snack. Instead you simply eat what you know works for you without any feelings of anxiety before you eat or sense of guilt after you eat.

As far as your personal growth and development is concerned, when you reach this point, you will have progressed through four distinct phases of learning a new skill. These four phases are categorized below. Knowledge of each of these four stages will help you consolidate your plan yet further, help you keep it intact for the future, and assist you when it comes to modelling your success with staying slim so you can apply your most effective behaviour strategies wherever else in life they may be of use to you.

Four stages of learning

UNCONSCIOUS INCOMPETENCE

Unconscious incompetence is the situation when something isn't working for you but you're not yet aware of the problem. This is the 'ignorance is bliss' stage. You have a food routine, but you're not really engaged in how it works or how it relates to the results you're looking for with your energy and your weight management.

For many people this stage of the learning process only lasts until a relatively early age in relation to weight management. This is the phase before weight and body image become a concern and in many societies nowadays, this blissful ignorance only lasts until the observation of parents, older siblings or friends discussing the merits of various food products, or thinking aloud about their weight and body shape eventually results in us thinking and behaving in the same way. Then we become aware of the media preoccupation with body image and this reinforces the notion that this is something we need to think about.

It's sad to say, but I've heard children, usually girls, as young as four and five making comments about 'naughty' foods and talking about being fat or thin. This is a clear example of modelling in action (though not in a good way) as these girls are simply copying what they have observed in their parents. It's also a good example of where beliefs will be formed; beliefs that can last for years and dictate many areas of these children's future.

CONSCIOUS INCOMPETENCE

Conscious incompetence is when you become aware that your current routine doesn't completely work for you. At this point, you'll be thinking about the steps you can take to rectify the situation by exploring your options, thinking about plans for change, building motivation and working out some strategies and solutions.

CONSCIOUS COMPETENCE

Conscious competence is when you have the solutions in place but you need to think hard about keeping on track with every aspect of them.

This is the stage where you need to be vigilant and flexible with your behaviour, and it helps to maintain focus on your ultimate objectives at all times.

UNCONSCIOUS COMPETENCE

Unconscious competence takes place when things are working for you without requiring a huge amount of effort to continue experiencing positive results. You have a tried and tested plan that achieves your desired results, and an integral part of this plan is the review and updating mechanisms that ensure you'll always continue to experience these results.

The foundations for ongoing success

When you have basic strategies that are successful, and an approach that is flexible, you can be confident that your healthy eating and weight management plan is designed for the long term. Remember that any challenges you face in the future are inevitable and are actually desirable in order that you can grow in confidence, knowing that your plan is built to last.

When you face a challenge, remain calm, pause for a moment and ask yourself what skills or knowledge you can apply in order to overcome the challenge. You are now fully equipped to stay slim for good and you are in control of your weight management. I wish you success and enjoyment of everything that success in this area will bring you.

Finally, just to keep you on track and motivated, here are a few examples of real-life situations where NLP techniques have played a crucial role in helping people stay slim for good.

Bullet-proof case studies: NLP and successful weight management in action

Bullet-proof solution 1: Let go of the past

Clare was in her late 40s when I met her, and one of the first things she said to me was that she had always struggled with her weight, ever since she was a young child, and had been following one type of diet or another since she was twelve.

As the discussions progressed, it transpired that Clare's relationship with her mother had been difficult, and for most of her formative years she had used food as a comfort when she felt things weren't going well. This began a cycle of binge eating, feelings of guilt, crash dieting, and sporadic bouts of intensive exercise. This had been the routine for over 40 years.

The first question to ask was if Clare was able to contemplate life being any other way. She had known this pattern for so long that it had become established as 'just the way things are'. Initially it was a novel concept for Clare to consider her life being any other way.

The next task was for Clare to decide how things were going to be different. She knew she didn't want to carry on as she was, but had never spent any time envisaging how things could be different in the long term. This part of our process took a little time because imagining a different future was a new concept for Clare. It was worth the effort though, as it helped her apply some context to what had in the past been a sequence of short-term, quick-fix behaviours.

This breakthrough helped Clare explore the specific behaviours she could try that would be different from the past and that would help her move towards the new future that she could now envisage. Next we worked on consolidating why she wanted to make this new future a reality. What was motivating about this new future? What difference would achieving it make to Clare's daily life?

Clare loved clothes and had worked in fashion at various stages of her career. Thinking about wearing more 'interesting' clothes, as she phrased, it was one thing that motivated her. Feeling more confident was also an attractive prospect but, as we dug a little deeper, it became apparent that one of the main drivers for future success was the idea that she could prove to herself there was another way to live; a life beyond the routines of the last 40 years. She wanted to be able to look back at this period of her life and say, 'I'm not that person any more. I've dealt with the things that used to make me miserable and moved on from them.'

(Contd)

From the moment Clare was able to create a visualization of herself in the future, looking back at her 'old' self in the past, she never looked back. She was able to add detail – sounds, smells, tastes and feelings – to her plans for the future and was then motivated to take consistent action every day that would move her closer to this outcome.

Having a new, clear and motivating plan for the future not only helped Clare to make choices that she was happier with on a day-to-day basis, but also became a great resource in times of stress that in the past would have driven her deeper into her familiar pattern of behaviour. Over the next few months, she faced a sequence of major challenges, a change in job, a relationship that came and went, the death of a pet and, the ultimate challenge, the death of her mother.

Keeping her end goal in mind helped Clare cope with all of these events, and with the passing of a little time she was soon able to acknowledge that she had become a different person and left her previous concerns behind.

How NLP helped Clare
Core beliefs, outcome planning, personal motivation, time line therapy, visualization, test and feedback review.

Bullet-proof solution 2: Model your own success

Anita was a successful media executive who had prioritized her career for a number of years. At the same time, she had suppressed her weight management goals. Her weight was always on her mind, but she took the view that she could address it at some later stage.

A number of years of eating erratically, grabbing meals and snacks on the go, drinking more alcohol than she felt she should and dealing with a stressful schedule had led to some extra kilos creeping on, and Anita was all too aware that her weekly routine consisted of work, stress, caffeine, sugar, alcohol, inconsistent eating, as well as lack of exercise and quality sleep. The question was, where to break into this cycle?

She decided that the first step would be to reintroduce exercise into her life. She had been sporty at school and had enjoyed keeping active in the early part of her career but had let this slip as work had become more demanding. Fortunately, this turned out to be an astute observation from Anita and this one change had an impact on every other area of her routine. Exercise helped her manage her stress, which helped her think more clearly through the working day. This helped her plan more time to take breaks to eat and this in turn allowed her to make choices with her meals and snacks that led to better energy and less sugary and fatty options. With more balanced blood sugar and energy levels, Anita found that she was better able to take on projects and activities at home in the evenings which meant she didn't automatically veer in the direction of the 'wind-down' wine as she called it and this in turn meant a better night of sleep leading to a better frame of mind for the following day.

Knowing the trigger behaviour that keeps everything else in place, and experiencing and reinforcing the positive energy and feelings that keep this trigger behaviour in place allows her to live with, means that Anita is always motivated to plan her exercise routines and make sure that they happen. They make the difference between living as she wants and living with compromise, as she felt she was for so many years. This means that exercise has now become non-negotiable.

How NLP helped Anita
Away from motivation, time line therapy, gut instinct, trigger behaviour, towards motivation, modelling.

Bullet-proof solution 3: Discover your higher purpose

Alan and Maria came to see me with a very familiar story. Both had been very fit and in great shape throughout their school years and university life, and had always kept each other on track with exercise and sports from when they met through to the time when they got married. Following their wedding, they both began to focus more on their careers and Alan took a job in a

(Contd)

location that meant he had a 75-minute commute either way from Monday to Friday. Because of the travel time, Alan began missing gym visits that he and Maria had planned together and, before long, Maria fell out of the habit of getting to the gym too.

In addition to his extended commute, Alan began to work longer hours, which meant he got home later and ate his evening meal later. At first Maria waited for Alan to eat but soon realized that she needed to eat earlier than 9pm or 10pm, so began to take her evening meal without him. Mealtimes, though, were the only time the couple got together so, in an attempt to have at least some quality time, Maria very soon fell into the routine of eating two meals each evening, her dinner by herself and then a second meal with Alan when he got home. Alan also ended up eating twice on many evenings when he would grab a snack and a drink on the train on his way home before eating dinner with Maria when he got in.

After a few months of this routine each of them was carrying an extra 14 kg to 21 kg (31 to 46 lb) and becoming increasingly unhappy with the situation. The tipping point for change came when they saw a photograph of themselves from a friend's wedding and were shocked at how heavy and unhealthy they looked. They had both been feeling progressively more lethargic and dejected at their lack of energy at times, and the photograph explained why.

Seeing the photograph was just the wake-up call they needed and their objectives at this point were simple. They both wanted to eat better, begin exercising again and boost their energy levels.

The first thing we did together was study the photograph that had got them to this point. This was the trigger event and a great 'away from' motivating factor, but I also asked Alan and Maria to pay some attention to what they wanted to motivate themselves towards. To begin with, they both struggled with this, so I asked them if they had experienced times in the past when they were working towards specific aims.

Both replied very quickly that they had and, in fact, always felt they were following a clear path until recently. They had both gone through school, university, then found their first jobs where they began to focus on promotion and career progression while at the same time allocating some time to socializing, finding a partner and then getting married. When asked what was next on the agenda, they both drew a blank and admitted that it felt as though they were drifting through each day at the moment and struggling with finding the time and energy to plan the future.

I challenged them to think a little bit more deeply about their daily routines and where their lives were heading. They responded by talking about the daily rewards, financial payback, satisfaction of a job well done, personal development and growth, and what they spend their money on. As they thought more about their future, they saw cars, holidays, homes, a nice lifestyle and eventually children.

I probed them a little more about the last item on the list. They both agreed that they wanted a family but not just yet, but because the notion of family life was a vague plan for the long-term future, it wasn't providing them with a clear enough context by which they could judge their current day-to-day life. As we worked to turn up the brightness on the concept of life with a young family and add in the sounds, smells, tastes and feelings of this new routine, Alan and Maria both agreed that their current situation was a long way from where they needed to be.

Alan knew that he didn't want to be working miles away, leaving so early and getting home so late that he didn't see the children, and Maria didn't want to be faced with the prospect of taking on the majority of the child care without assistance, particularly if she felt as though she didn't have enough energy to deal with everything on her own agenda already. More urgently, even though they weren't planning on having children immediately, Maria knew that she wanted to be in good shape when they got round to starting the family, and was hoping to feel good throughout her pregnancy.

When I asked if their current eating patterns were ones that were in keeping with the future they visualized for themselves with their

(Contd)

family, the answer was obvious. Once Alan and Maria had put their food routine into the context of what they wanted for the future, it was far easier to highlight where they could make changes now and also much simpler to follow patterns of behaviour that were consistent with where they wanted to get to. Food and drink had simply become comforts in a busy routine, and there was very little engagement from either of them as to how they were behaving and the results this behaviour was leading them to. With new clarity on how healthy eating, and exercise, fitted into the master plan of their lives, and an understanding of how decisions in these areas could make a huge difference to their ability to perform in other areas, specifically their role as parents, Alan and Maria were motivated to change their routine.

It took five months for Alan and eight months for Maria, but within this time they were both back to the physical shape they wanted to be in and felt much better energy throughout each day. Alan embarked on the hunt for a new job closer to home and Maria had arranged to work from home two days a week to help her plan their home life a little bit better and to begin the initial preparations for life as a family.

How NLP helped Alan and Maria
Trigger event, motivating factors, chunking up, reframing, submodalities, outcome planning.

Bullet-proof solution 4: Get out of your own way

Consider the following opening dialogue I had with someone who voluntarily attended a nutrition clinic for a consultation.

Me: Hello, how are you, how can I help?

Debbie: Hi. I wanted to come and talk to you. I need to lose weight but nothing seems to work for me. I've tried Weight Watchers in the past, and Rosemary Connelly, but I find the plans really difficult to follow because they don't include any food that I like. I can't eat breakfast and I don't really like fruit, or vegetables and I don't really like to eat much in the way of carbohydrates. I've never been a fan of red meat. It's really difficult for me to eat healthily in the daytime because there's nothing good to eat in the office. You can ask anyone, they all know how hard I try but how much I struggle with finding the right thing to eat.

What became clear very early on in this meeting was that Debbie was still at the stage where she would rather focus on her perceived problems rather than solutions. She wasn't aware of it, and she probably would have denied it, but she was comforted by and almost enjoying all the reasons why she wasn't able to achieve what she said she wanted to achieve. She had even carved out a reputation based on her 'struggle' with eating well. Everyone knew about her food dislikes and she enjoyed talking about her situation whenever she could.

None of the discussions that Debbie had, internally or externally, included anything close to a plan for success. They were always about why success was impossible for her. Yet she was insistent when questioned about her commitment to losing weight. She was adamant that it was one of her top priorities.

I wished I'd had a tape recorder to illustrate to Debbie the internal struggle clearly being verbalized. On the one side, her purported desire to lose weight; on the other, all the great reasons why losing weight never worked. The difficulty for Debbie was that the internal conversation was so familiar to her there was never any new insight on the situation. Discussions with her friends, colleagues, and even me to begin with, simply reinforced her belief that, no matter what people suggested, or what worked for other people, she was different by virtue of the fact that none of the solutions that worked for other people would work for her. She tried to use this difference to help her stand out from the crowd. If she could have heard how incongruent her conversation was and how negative the net result came across as, I'm convinced she would have changed her tune.

Clearly we needed to change Debbie's view of her situation. I'm not sure that she, as an intelligent, articulate, resourceful individual,

(Contd)

would have accepted the statements she herself was making, had they been coming from someone else, so I simply made the comment that if she had tried so many previous plans and approaches in the past and was so clear on what didn't work and what she didn't like, she must now be pretty close to putting the final touches to the plan that is perfect for her.

For a moment she paused. I could almost see her shift physically as the weight of responsibility for her eating habits landed back in her lap. For years she had been passing this responsibility to other people: to the designers of the various weight loss plans she had followed but that hadn't worked for her; to the buyers at all manner of supermarkets and shops that only stocked foods she didn't like and couldn't eat; to the company responsible for the catering at her office; to any number of people, none of whom had any knowledge of or interest in Debbie's weight.

Ultimately, the only person who really cared about Debbie's weight was Debbie. The only person who could make the necessary changes was Debbie. Only when she was able to shift her attention away from the importance of justifying why she couldn't get the result she wanted and onto considering everything required in order to get the right result, did she stand any chance of success. Once she was reminded of this, we agreed three simple tasks for her to be getting on with.

She was to make a list of all the foods she liked and that she could eat, and come up with as many meal and snack options as she could using these items.

Each time she found herself thinking or verbalizing a reason why she couldn't eat healthily, she was to write it down and next to it write down a counter argument, an option or a solution.

Without mentioning the Meta Model, we agreed that Debbie would stop generalizing, distorting and deleting to come up with general reasons why she couldn't lose weight, and begin focusing on specific reasons why she was going to lose weight.

Within six weeks Debbie had lost a few kilos. She was a little disappointed with this, which told me that we still had some work to do, but when I pointed out that her weight was now moving in the right direction and that she clearly had some success strategies to build on, she was more able to acknowledge what she had achieved and able to accept that she had taken a big step forward on the road to weight loss success.

Phase two of Debbie's progress was simple. Until this point she still believed that her attitude to food – her likes and mainly dislikes – was something that gave her a personality; something that made her stand out and get attention. By working with submodalities to shrink down Debbie's experiences and visualizations of herself as someone who gets attention because they have specific dietary requirements, and then enhancing the submodalities of the notion of Debbie getting lots of attention because she had managed to lose weight, we were able to break through the issues that had prevented Debbie from making progress to date.

How NLP helped Debbie
Belief change, inner dialogue, the Meta Model, reframing, submodalities.

Bullet-proof solution 5: Slow down to speed up your results

If you still have reservations around the benefits of a more thoughtful approach to weight loss, here's an example of precisely how this approach was employed to overcome 20 years worth of frustration and unhappiness with yo-yo dieting.

Amanda's weight had always fluctuated. Beginning when she was 17, she followed a variety of 'crash diets' and at one point her weight dropped as low as 42 kg (93 lb). The heaviest she got was when she crept up to 68 kg (150 lb) at the time of her university graduation. Her weight settled around 63 kg (139 lb) for the next ten years, though Amanda admits to never being happy with this. When she got married, she dropped to 60 kg (132 lb) through cutting down on carbohydrates and exercising with a combination of cardiovascular workouts and strength training.

(Contd)

Although Amanda was extremely dissatisfied with the way she looked, she never seemed quite able to get her weight under control. She just didn't seem to have the time. For 17 years, work was always a higher priority as she focused on a fast-paced, highly stressful career with lots of travelling and client entertaining which played havoc with her food regime. She ended up eating lots of rich food at mealtimes, in larger quantities than were necessary, and then surviving on carbohydrates and sugary snacks between meals in the hope this would keep up her energy levels.

The one thing that finally broke the cycle for Amanda was becoming pregnant. She was overjoyed to have two children within a couple of years, but couldn't resist keeping a close eye on how this was affecting her weight, which fluctuated from under 70 kg (154 lb) prior to her first pregnancy to peak at just over 84 kg (185 lb) during each of her pregnancies.

Following the birth of her second child, Amanda spent much of the next 18 months becoming increasingly miserable with her body shape as her weight hovered once again around the 68 kg (150 lb). She felt she'd returned back to where she was at her heaviest during her university days. During this period, she took advice on exercise and through this managed to improve her fitness and strength levels. Still something was missing when it came to feeling motivated to make changes to what she was eating. Amanda was well aware of what she should do with regard to making simple changes to her diet, but never felt motivated to put these changes into practice.

Then, everything changed. A few cheeky comments about her shape from family members sparked a level of emotion that hadn't existed before. Amanda felt increasingly frustrated that she'd got herself into a position where people felt they could comment, openly and negatively, on the way she looked. And one thing in particular marked the beginning of something new. Her three-year-old son pointed out and grabbed hold of some of Amanda's 'fleshy bits' that she disliked so much. This really depressed her, but was enough to kick-start her into doing something about her situation.

At this point, it all came together for Amanda. She realized just how miserable she was with herself but, more than that, she finally accepted that she just couldn't go on like this. She felt that from this moment onwards, she had no excuses for not fixing her situation.

She knew she had a good understanding of nutrition and what she should be eating, and she knew that she had all the information on exercise that anyone could ever need to make a difference to their body. She now felt there was no good reason why she shouldn't be acting on what she knew. She decided there and then that it was up to her to just get on with it.

She thought about what had hindered her in the past. The main barrier to success that she could think of was that she always had unrealistic goals for herself, the favourite of which was to aim to lose 3 kg (7 lb) in a single week. Whenever she set herself this goal, she would start starving herself for as long as possible and then, by day four or five, be driven by a frenzy to feast on chocolate, then be really fed up with herself, tell herself she had 'failed again' and vow to start again next Monday!

This time she was determined not to repeat the same mistakes of the past. She decided to start with a slightly longer-term plan, and drew up a schedule for the next six weeks on the calendar. The schedule contained all-important dates such as a wedding anniversary and any special parties or occasions. She then set a goal of losing 6 kg (13 lb) in six weeks. She broke this goal down even further so that she'd be aiming to lose 1 kg (2 lb) in week one and then 1 kg (2 lb) during each subsequent week. Amanda decided she would weigh herself each Monday morning and if she had achieved her weekly goal, she would reward herself with a 'treat' such as a new shirt, a belt, a manicure or some earrings – not something related to eating.

Amanda also forced herself to write down everything that she ate and drank every day in her food diary. She admitted to thinking this tedious to begin with, but then found it really useful to look back over each week, think about what she had consumed and how this had affected her energy levels on various days. She credits the food diary with teaching her how to examine her diet over a longer period and avoid the pitfalls of chocolate bars for the first time in her life.

(Contd)

The results were dramatic. Amanda managed to drop 6 kg (13 lb) during her first six-week schedule. She then dropped an additional 4 kg (9 lb) with her second six-week plan. Buoyed by this success she went on to devise further six-week schedules designed to maintain her weight precisely where she had managed to get it and where she wanted it to stay.

For the first few weeks, Amanda was working through a back injury and so did a limited amount of exercise. From week four onwards she gradually increased her activity with a combination of running, strength training, yoga and hiking, usually managing some form of activity three or four times a week.

Amanda credits her success with not making changes to her diet that were too drastic. She cut out chocolate and reduced her wine consumption to a maximum of four glasses a week. By using her diary, she worked out that keeping off the carbohydrates after lunch time, increasing her water consumption, and increasing her daily fruit and vegetable portions all worked extremely well and gave her the results she'd always been looking for.

One of the biggest benefits that Amanda reports is that the great thing about where she is now is, apart from feeling lighter, fitter, healthier and happier, all of which are great on their own, she also feels 'empowered'. She had always secretly hated that word but now uses it to sum up the feeling of having taken charge and finally made a breakthrough with something that had been such a large part of her life for such a long time.

How NLP helped Amanda
Trigger moment, no failure only feedback, outcome planning, chunking, context.

Further reading

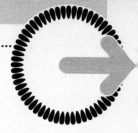

Archer, J., *Be Your Own Life Coach* (Hodder Education, 2010)

Atkinson, Dr. M. and Bailey, C., *The Intelligent Way to Lose Weight: A Revolutionary Personalised Approach to Healthy Weight Loss* (Berlin, Another Country Publishing)

Bavister, S. and Vickers, A., *Essential NLP* (Hodder Education, 2010)

James, T. and Woodsmall, W., *Time Line Therapy and the Basis of Personality* (Meta Publications, 1989)

Jenner, P., *Transform Your Life with NLP* (Hodder Education, 2010)

O'Connor, J. and Seymour, J., *Introducing NLP: Psychological Skills for Understanding and Influencing People* (Conari Press, 2011)

Lewis, B. and Pucelik, F., *Magic of NLP Demystified: A Pragmatic Guide to Communication & Change* (Metamorphous Press, 1990)

Robbins, A., *Unlimited Power: The New Science of Personal Achievement* (Pocket Books, 2001)

Index

Image credits